HISTORY OF THE EUROPEAN ASSOCIATION FOR HAEMATOPATHOLOGY

KARL LENNERT

HISTORY OF THE EUROPEAN ASSOCIATION FOR HAEMATOPATHOLOGY

TRANSLATED BY MARTHA SOEHRING

Springer

Prof. em. Dr. med. Dr. h.c. mult. Karl Lennert
Niemannsweg 26
24105 Kiel, Germany
Formerly:
Director, Institute of Pathology
University of Kiel
24105 Kiel, Germany

ISBN-10 3-540-34886-7 Springer Berlin Heidelberg New York
ISBN-13 978-3-540-34886-3 Springer Berlin Heidelberg New York

Library of Congress Control Number: 2006926722

Springer is a part of Springer Science+Business Media
springer.com

Editor: Gabriele Schröder, Heidelberg
Desk Editor: Ellen Blasig, Heidelberg
Cover design: Frido Steinen-Broo, EStudio Calamar, Spain
Typesetting and production: LE-T_EX Jelonek, Schmidt&Vöckler GbR, Leipzig, Germany

Printed on acid-free paper 27/3100/YL 5 4 3 2 1 0

PREFACE

During the last quarter of the 20th century a paradigmatic change occurred in the understanding and classification of malignant lymphomas. This was primarily a result of the discovery of the two lymphocyte systems (the B-cell and T-cell systems with numerous variants), which was made possible mainly through the use of many antibodies, most of which were monoclonal. In order to distinguish the various types of lymphoma it is necessary to use an optimum technique that allows recognition of the same cell types in both imprints and sections. The pioneer work of A. A. MAXIMOW more than 100 years ago laid the basis for developing such a technique for preparing sections and imprints of high quality, which are a prerequisite for both exact morphological diagnoses and the application of antibodies. This led to the development of new classifications that also proved to be largely valid when tested with recent molecular genetic techniques.

The development began in Europe in 1972 and soon led to the systematic application of a new lymphoma classification, which was proposed by the members of the European Lymphoma Club at a meeting in Kiel, Germany (thus the name "Kiel classification") in 1974. The classification quickly came into widespread use in Europe. In the USA (and institutions dependent on the USA), however, the classification met with great resistance and opposition. Finally, a breakthrough occurred after an international study suggested by Dr. J.O. ARMITAGE and performed by a group of true lymphoma experts (pathologists); the overwhelming results of this study were presented by Dr. S.A. ROSENBERG in Omaha, NE, USA in 1997.

Since the USA-dominated Society for Hematopathology was not interested in establishing a separate section for the large group of European haematopathologists, the European Association for Haematopathology was founded in 1988. The Association has developed into an effective organization with a steadily growing number of members (from 246 in 1988 to more than 500 registered participants at the last congress in Thessaloniki, Greece).

The author has been asked many times to write a chronicle of these developments. On the one hand, it was a pleasure to accept – for the sake of a good cause. On the other hand, there were several difficulties. First, I had to rely mostly on notes taken in my own diary; I was well aware of the risk that the report would be too personal. Second, it was difficult to give due honour to the many colleagues involved and to mention them all in the report. It felt awkward to write "I" so many times, knowing that none of the studies would have been possible without the participation of colleagues, especially co-workers at the Institute of Pathology in Kiel. I thank them all for their patience, cooperation, and loyalty. Of my many co-workers there are four who deserve special mention, namely, Professor E. Kaiserling, Professor H. K. Müller-Hermelink, Professor E. W. Schwarze, and Professor H. Stein. I am also grateful to my loyal clinical colleague Professor G. Brittinger and his large group of clinicians, who readily provided biopsy material and clinical data even under difficult conditions. In order to obtain the material the local pathologists had to give their consent, and they did so generously. The concepts underlying the Kiel classification were scrutinized in immunological studies done by members of a "special research area" (sponsored by the German Research Foundation), of which Professor W. Müller-Ruchholtz was co-chairman; he was a crucial critical partner. The harmonious cooperation within the European Lymphoma Club was of great value, and I could always rely on the members' support. My thanks are also due to the medical technicians at the Institute in Kiel; when I examined the slides they had prepared I was often spurred on by their excellent skills (e.g. Giemsa staining).

This report would not have been possible without the energetic support of the President of the European Association for Haematopathology, Dr. M. A. Piris, and the Treasurer, Professor J. H. J. M. van Krieken. They spontaneously agreed to have the Association cover the costs of publication. As with earlier books, I am also very grateful to Mrs. M. Soehring for her prudent and constructive support while translating the text.

It was a pleasure to work with Ms. G. Schröder und Ms. E. Blasig of Springer-Verlag, whose competent and untiring efforts made it possible to publish this report in time for the next congress of the European Association for Haematopathology in Vienna, Austria.

Kiel, May 2006 Karl Lennert

FOREWORD

The European Association for Haematopathology (EAHP) was created with the aim of integrating lymphoma basic and clinical research, stemming from the deeply held conviction that only by pursuing research into clinical translation will we eventually be able to refine lymphoma diagnostic categories. This will make it possible for us to develop new diagnostic and therapeutic tools, using more efficiently the therapies that are currently available. The work of the EAHP and the Society of Hematopathology created the basis for the REAL Classification that finally, under the sponsorship of the WHO, led to the publication of the unique WHO Lymphoma Classification that is now recognized throughout the world. The efforts to promote a lymphoma classification with a solid biological foundation is described in this extraordinary book, in which Professor K. Lennert narrates his memories of those years and of the work that was so infused with his strength of purpose and dedication.

Many of today's young clinicians and researchers will find it difficult to appreciate the damage that the confusion concerning lymphoma classification wrought on patients suffering from lymphoproliferative conditions during the period related here. Professor Lennert's personal recollections describe the formula by which this crisis was overcome – the integration of basic and clinical research in enthusiastically conducted work directed towards well-chosen ends. This formula has been adopted by leading pathologists in Europe and the USA, so ensuring that the Lymphoma Classification will continue to be kept up to date. Indeed, this synthesis of fundamental and applied research has become the model of choice, replicated by other scientific societies throughout the clinical world.

The fruits of Professor Lennert's scientific career and objectives are now embodied within the WHO Lymphoma Classification. This fully embraces the main proposals of the Kiel Classification, the establishment of tumoral categories that integrate cell lineage, stage of differentiation, molecular markers and diagnostic morphological features. As such, it provides haematopathologists and clinicians with a reliable tool for the accurate identification of the different lymphoma types.

While the European Association for Haematopathology was created during the era described in this book, it remains an exemplary pathology society, open to basic and clinical researchers, and currently has around 500 members worldwide. Today it represents the natural continuation of the spirit that in the 1970s and 1980s pervaded the Institute of Pathology in Kiel. It was there that Professor Lennert was host to dozens of haematopathologists from all over the world, and where he provided them with an opportunity to share projects, exchange ideas and compare results. This contributed greatly to establishing the community as we know it today, with its freedom from international boundaries.

In recognition of all this, we take great pleasure in writing this foreword to Professor Lennert's memoirs and welcome the publication of this book to mark the occasion of his 85th birthday.

Dr. Miguel A Piris	Prof. Stefano Pileri
President EAHP	President Elect EAHP

CONTENTS

1	Introduction	1
2	Classification of Malignant Lymphomas	5
2.1	1958–1971	5
2.2	The WHO Classification I (1968–1976)	6
2.3	Lymphocyte Transformation and the B-Cell and T-Cell Systems. Initial Immunochemical Studies, 1971–1972	8
2.4	The Kiel Lymphoma Study Group	11
2.5	1972–1973	14
2.6	Prelude to European Cooperation, 1973	14
2.7	The European Lymphoma Club (ELC)	17
2.8	The Kiel Classification, 1974	18
2.9	Presentation of the Kiel Classification, 1974–1980	25
2.9.1	Vienna, Austria, 29–31 August 1974	26
2.9.2	London, UK, 24–28 August 1975	26
2.9.3	Bad Nauheim, Germany, 29 September – 1 October 1975	27
2.9.4	Vienna, 6–11 October and 14 November 1975	27
2.9.5	Damp, Germany, 3–8 November 1975	28
2.9.6	Jerusalem, Israel, 17–31 March 1976	28
2.9.7	Spain, 23–25 September 1976 and 21–22 October 1978	29
2.9.8	Boston, MA, USA, 15 October 1976	29
2.9.9	Washington, DC, USA, 17–21 October 1976	30
2.9.10	Brazil, 25–29 October 1976	31
2.9.11	Japan, 2–8 April 1977	32
2.9.12	Brussels, Belgium, 14 May 1977	33
2.9.13	Bucharest, Rumania, 25–27 May 1977	34
2.9.14	Cold Spring Harbor, NY, USA, 7–12 September 1977	35
2.9.15	Chicago, IL and Winston-Salem, NC, USA, 18–22 September 1977	36
2.9.16	Rochester, MN, USA, 1–3 October 1977	36
2.9.17	Munich, Germany, 16–18 June 1978	37
2.9.18	Poland, 9–12 October 1978	37
2.9.19	Thessaloniki, Greece, 16–17 October 1978	39
2.9.20	Lisbon, Portugal, 27–30 January 1980	39
2.9.21	New York, NY, USA, 2–8 March 1980	39
2.9.22	Paris, France, 15–19 September 1980	40
2.10	Other Means of Dissemination of the Kiel Classification	41

2.10.1 Establishment of Research Centres and Study Groups 41
2.10.2 Major Publications 41
2.11 Clinical Relevance of the Kiel Classification 42
2.12 Genetic and Molecular Genetic Studies 43
2.13 A Sideline: Gastrointestinal Lymphomas in Tunisia, 11–15 December 1978 44
2.14 Attempts to Agree on a Universal Classification of Malignant Lymphoma, 1974–1982 46
2.14.1 Florence, Italy, 20–26 October 1974 47
2.14.2 Warrenton, VA, USA, 4–5 September 1975 47
2.14.3 Villejuif, France, 20–25 June 1977 50
2.14.4 Geneva, 1–5 May 1978 50
2.14.5 The NCI Study, 1975–1980 52
2.14.5.1 Tour of the Institutions Involved in the NCI Study 54
2.14.5.2 Evaluation of the Results of the NCI Study 55
2.14.6 Presentation of the Working Formulation, 1982 56
2.15 Comparison of the Lukes-Collins Classification and the Kiel Classification 61
2.15.1 Washington, DC, 20 October 1976 63
2.15.2 Stockholm, Sweden, 29–31 March 1979 63
2.15.3 Noordwijkerhout, The Netherlands, 3–6 April 1979 63
2.15.4 Athens, Greece, 6–10 April 1981 65
2.15.5 Kiel, Germany, 16–21 April 1981 67
2.16 Acceptance of the Kiel Classification, 1981–1987 68
2.16.1 Vienna, 15–18 February 1981 68
2.16.2 Ljubljana, Yugoslavia, 14–15 April 1981 69
2.16.3 Erice, Sicily, 3–9 May 1981 70
2.16.4 Erfurt, Germany, 13 May 1981 70
2.16.5 Montreal, Canada, 17–21 September 1981 70
2.16.6 Jerusalem, 22–25 September 1981 71
2.16.7 Kiel, 7–9 October 1981 72
2.16.8 Oxford, UK, 25–30 January 1982 72
2.16.9 USA, 25 February – 5 March 1982 75
2.16.10 Copenhagen, Denmark, 28–30 June 1982 77
2.16.11 Freiburg, Germany, 6 July 1982 78
2.16.12 Kiel, 2–6 August 1982 78
2.16.13 Seattle, WA, USA, 6–7 September 1982 79
2.16.14 Birmingham, UK, 20 September 1982 80
2.16.15 Brazil, 22–26 September 1982 81
2.16.16 Rome, Italy, 3–6 October 1982 84
2.16.17 1983 84
2.16.17.1 Wiesbaden, Germany, 14 April 1983 84

2.16.17.2	Lucerne, Switzerland, 24–28 May 1983	85
2.16.17.3	Kiel, 5–11 September 1983	85
2.16.17.4	Cold Spring Harbor, NY, USA, 14–15 September 1983	86
2.16.17.5	Hamburg, Germany, 19–24 September 1983	87
2.16.17.6	London, 29–30 September 1983	87
2.16.17.7	Kiel, 1–7 October 1983	87
2.16.17.8	Bologna, Italy, 17–18 October 1983	87
2.16.17.9	Morocco, 23–26 October 1983	88
2.16.18	1984	88
2.16.18.1	France, 26–28 April 1984	88
2.16.18.2	China, 29 April – 12 May 1984	89
2.16.18.3	Japan, 12–19 May 1984	94
2.16.18.4	Siena, Italy, 24–26 May 1984	96
2.16.18.5	Kiel, 24–27 June 1984	96
2.16.18.6	Buenos Aires, Argentina, 2–4 September 1984	96
2.16.18.7	USA, 5–22 September 1984	97
2.16.18.8	UK, 18–21 November 1984	99
2.16.19	1985	100
2.16.19.1	Puerto de la Cruz, Tenerife, 8–10 March 1985	100
2.16.19.2	Kiel, 24–30 April 1985	101
2.16.19.3	Stockholm, Sweden, 6 June 1985	101
2.16.19.4	Kiel, 10–11 June 1985	101
2.16.19.5	Prague, Czechoslovakia, 3–6 September 1985	101
2.16.19.6	Kiel, 13–15 September 1985	102
2.16.19.7	Athens, 4–5 October 1985	102
2.16.19.8	Vienna, 6–9 October 1985	103
2.16.20	Attempts to Form a European-American Alliance, 1986	103
2.16.20.1	Kiel, 26–28 January 1986	103
2.16.20.2	New Orleans, LA, USA, 8–12 March 1986	103
2.16.20.3	After-Effects, April 1986	106
2.16.20.4	Founding of the Society for Hematopathology in Retrospect	108
2.16.21	Further Events, 1986–1987	109
2.16.21.1	April–July 1986	109
2.16.21.2	Vienna, 27 August – 5 September 1986	109
2.16.21.3	Far East, 22 September – 7 October 1986	110
2.16.21.4	Chicago, 7–12 March 1987	110
2.16.21.5	Garden City, Long Island, NY, USA, 13–14 March 1987	111
2.16.21.6	Boston, MA, 15–17 March 1987	111
2.16.21.7	Oberhausen, Germany, 23 March – 7 April 1987	111
2.17	Founding of the European Lymphoma Study Group	112
2.17.1	Kiel, 7–8 November 1980	112

2.17.2 Kiel, 20–24 October 1981 113
2.17.3 Southampton, UK, 25–28 September 1983 115
2.17.4 Toulouse, France, 1–3 April 1985 116
2.17.5 Brussels, 27–29 October 1986 116
2.17.6 Geneva, 14–15 March 1988 116
3 Founding of the European Association for Haematopathology 117
3.1 Prelude, 1986–1988 117
3.1.1 Kiel, 9–11 December 1987 117
3.1.2 Kiel, 17–19 February 1988 118
3.1.3 21 March 1988 118
3.2 Geneva, 11–15 April 1988 119
3.3 Porto, Portugal, 6–7 September 1989 122
4 Epilogue, 1989–2004 123
References 125

1 INTRODUCTION

Haematology, the science of the blood and its diseases, was a purely clinical domain for a long time, because diseases of the blood could usually be diagnosed on blood or bone marrow smears. Haematopathology, on the other hand, is generally based on changes in the micro- or macroscopic appearance of blood-forming organs; a haematopathological diagnosis mostly depends on a histological examination. It took a long time before clinicians (at least in Europe) gave up their hegemony and allowed pathologists to have a say. A good example was the public debate between A. A. Maximow [1] (Fig. 1), the first haematopathologist of any stature, and O. Naegeli, an internist from Zurich, Switzerland, who accused pathologists of complete incompetence in diagnostic haematology [2] and was applauded by clinical haematologists. Maximow was at a great advantage, however, because he could identify blood and bone marrow cells not only in smears, with which clinicians were familiar, but also in histological sections prepared from bone marrow biopsies. The latter made it possible for him to use an optimum technique. He embedded the biopsy tissue in resin from which he cut ultrathin sections, which he stained with azure II-eosin; later he added haematoxylin to the staining. Furthermore, Maximow was blessed with the ability to reproduce exactly what he had seen under the microscope in water colour paintings. Hence it was possible to learn to make haematological diagnoses on sections and smears from his illustrations.

After the death of Maximow in 1928, his work was carried on at the Institute of Anatomy in Chicago, IL, USA by his successor W. Bloom, whom M. H. Block considered to be his real teacher [3]. In Germany J. Wienbeck started using Maximow's technique during World War II [4]. Unfortunately, his studies were halted by his sudden death. In 1945 I began using Maximow's technique and taught myself to apply it in the study of bone marrow and lymph nodes by reading Maximow's comprehensive description in the handbook edited by P. Stöhr and W. von Möllendorff [1], which was of excellent didactic quality [5]. Instead of azure II-eosin it soon became evident that the Giemsa solution produced by Merck (Darmstadt, Germany) was just as good and much easier to use. Good embedding in paraffin proved to be sufficient for routine diagnoses. Re-embedding in resin (JB-4; the method is described in [6]) was performed in special studies, e.g. analyses of high-grade malignant B-cell lymphomas [7] or of T-cell lymphoma variants.

MAXIMOW's pioneer studies were the impulse for the albeit hesitant development of the field of haematopathology. The reader may refer to the review of R. F. DORFMAN in his MAUD ABBOTT Lecture in 1994 [8] for more information about research in this field and also to the brilliant book written by M. M. WINTROBE [9] who competently described the research of most of the haematologists all over the world.

In the USA two research centres were established by H. RAPPAPORT and R. J. LUKES. Their work culminated in two atlases published by the Armed Forces Institute of Pathology [10,11]. In Europe A. H. T. ROBB-SMITH founded the first lymph node registry in 1947 [12]. In 1978 W.St.C. SYMMERS gave the first monographic description of the pathology of lymphoreticular tissue [13].

There are now several societies that were specifically founded to promote the field of haematopathology. The first was the **Japan Society of the Reticuloendothelial System**, founded in Tokyo, Japan in 1960. Its first president was K. AKAZAKI and the first vice-president was S. YAMAGATA. The term "reticuloendothelial system" (RES), which was originally coined by L. ASCHOFF and co-workers, included all of haematology, including haematopathology. The first published proceedings of the first general meeting in Sendai, Japan in 1961 focussed on morphological and functional studies of the RES [14]. As time went by the proceedings contained more and more clinical and pathological-anatomical studies in the whole field of haematology. Nevertheless, haematopathology continued to be the main focus. In the first eight years the number of members rose to more than 1,000.

In 1981 the **Society for Hematopathology** was founded in the USA. Its first president was C. W. BERARD and the first vice-president was DORFMAN. More about this Society will be presented in a later chapter (see p. 108).

The following report will tell the history of the third haematological society, known as the **European Association for Haematopathology**.

In haematopathology nowadays both the practical and the scientific interest is focussed mainly on two subjects, namely, the pathology of myeloproliferative disorders and malignant lymphomas. In the following I shall concentrate on the pathology of malignant lymphomas.

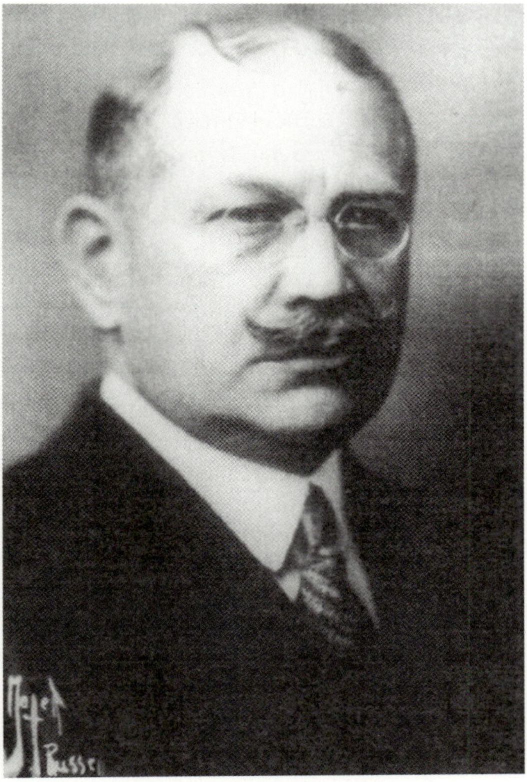

Fig. 1 A. MAXIMOW, Etron, 1917 (photograph kindly provided by R. DEYEV, Saint Petersburg, Russia)

2 CLASSIFICATION OF MALIGNANT LYMPHOMAS

2.1 1958–1971

A. RÜTTIMANN [15] invited LUKES and myself to present the American and European concepts of lymphoma classification at the International Symposium on Lymphology in **Zurich** in 1966. This was a simple task for LUKES [16], because he could fall back on the concept of E. A. GALL and T. B. MALLORY [17], which was later modified by RAPPAPORT [9,18] and accepted everywhere in the United States. On the basis of analyses of haematoxylin and eosin (H&E) stained sections RAPPAPORT distinguished six cytological types of lymphoma, each of which could show a nodular or diffuse growth pattern. Hodgkin's disease was included in this concept. On the whole, LUKES accepted RAPPAPORT's concept, but did not want to include the "mixed (lymphocytic-histiocytic) type". He also questioned the inclusion of Hodgkin's disease because its nature had not yet been clarified. LUKES presented this as the American concept, but emphasized that it would be necessary to add to the basic lymphoma entities on the basis of further parameters.

It was not so easy for me to demonstrate a European concept of lymphoma classification [19], because at the time there was no such thing. My sympathies were with the concept of ROBB-SMITH [20], who was convinced that it was widely recognized in Europe. He distinguished reactive hyperplasias, progressive hyperplasias (e.g. chronic lymphocytic leukaemia) and sarcomas of lymphatic tissue.

At the Institute of Pathology in Kiel we used not only H&E staining but also Giemsa-stained sections for a cytological classification. We also applied histochemical methods and performed electron microscopic investigations, even on formalin-fixed tissue. It became evident that the tumour cells of some of the so-called reticulosarcomas contained a large amount of rough endoplasmic reticulum. The cells in such cases were thus interpreted as immunoblasts. At the Symposium in Zurich I demonstrated a typical case of this type and proposed the term "immunoblastic sarcoma". The entities that we could recognize at the time were presented in a table. These included some entities that were not recognizable in the American concept, e.g. chronic lymphocytic leukaemia, lymphosarcoma, Waldenström's macroglobulinaemia and generalized giant follicular hyperplasia (Brill-Symmers' disease).

2.2 THE WHO CLASSIFICATION I (1968–1976)

It was evident that consensus on a generally accepted classification of malignant lymphomas was urgently needed. As a representative of the World Health Organization (WHO), H. Torloni tried to organize the pubilication of a "Blue Book" on these neoplasms. He invited G. Mathé, G. T. O'Conor

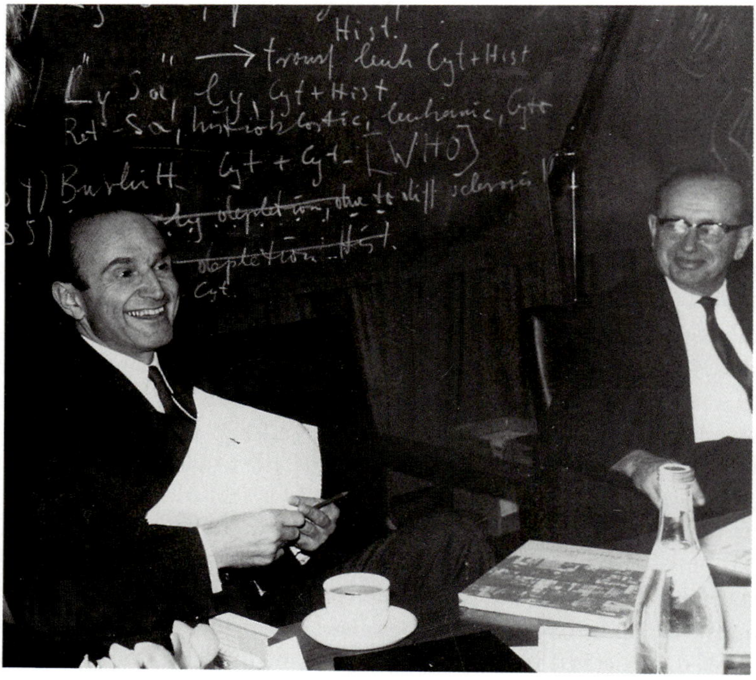

Fig. 2 Workshop to prepare the first WHO classification in Kiel, Germany, 1968. *Left*: G. Mathé. *Right*: H. Rappaport

and RAPPAPORT (Fig. 2) to the Institute of Pathology in **Kiel, Germany** in 1968 (18–22 November). I was to be the host and a participant in the discussion. There was a lively and controversial debate. MATHÉ defended RAPPAPORT's concept of the cytological diversity of nodular (follicular) lymphomas, whereas I held the view that only one group of tumour cells proliferates in follicular lymphomas, namely, germinal centre cells. The debate escalated as the days went by, until MATHÉ suddenly gave in and agreed that follicular lymphoma should be considered a single entity. The resulting lymphoma classification did not conform to the American concept originally favoured by MATHÉ. We also discussed at length the possibilities offered by cytochemistry in the diagnosis of leukaemia, as presented to the group by my co-worker L. D. LEDER. Over the next four years, however, I did not hear anything more about a manuscript.

At the beginning of 1972 the participants each received a copy of the final "Blue Book" manuscript. It was a big surprise, because the results of the discussion in Kiel were not mentioned at all. For example, follicular lymphoma was not defined as a single entity in the classification of malignant lymphomas. Therefore I asked MATHÉ to add a footnote to the classification table stating that I did not wish to be identified with the WHO classification. Since MATHÉ refused to do so, I asked to have my name deleted from the list of editors. R. GÉRARD-MARCHANT also reacted by having his name deleted, especially since the lymphoma classification proposed by MATHÉ and RAPPAPORT had not been negotiated with the other members of the group.

A year later RAPPAPORT presented the WHO classification at a workshop in **Chicago** (see p. 14). There was a very lively discussion following his report and then a vote. Only about 50% of the participants voted "Yes", approx. 25% voted "No" and the rest abstained.

In September 1975 TORLONI's successor at the WHO in Geneva, Switzerland, L.H. SOBIN, corresponded with MATHÉ and myself. I was still supposed to be a member of the board of editors of the "Blue Book", but I asked to be removed from the list.

In December 1975 the members of the European Lymphoma Club (ELC, see p. 17) wrote a letter to SOBIN declaring their unanimous opinion that the proposed WHO Classification was not acceptable and that they would not recommend its use. Other letters protesting the classification were written to MATHÉ by GÉRARD-MARCHANT and D. A. G. GALTON. Nevertheless MATHÉ and RAPPAPORT published the "Blue Book" in 1976 in collaboration with O'CONOR and TORLONI without any significant changes [21]. MATHÉ also presented the WHO Classification at a meeting of the International Academy of Pathology in **Washington, DC, USA** that same year. The classification was out of date before it was even published. As far as I know, it was never used except at a few hospitals (e.g. in Moscow and Tokyo).

2.3 LYMPHOCYTE TRANSFORMATION AND THE B-CELL AND T-CELL SYSTEMS. INITIAL IMMUNOCHEMICAL STUDIES, 1971–1972

At earlier international meetings I had already stated the view that follicular lymphomas are proliferations *only* of germinal centre cells ("germinoblasts" and "germinocytes") that had already been identified in normal lymph nodes. One of these occasions was the first meeting of the European Division of the International Society of Haematology in **Milan, Italy** in 1971 (5–11 September) [22]. There, at a cocktail party, A. Stacher approached me and asked me to give a lecture on malignant lymphomas (later called "non-Hodgkin's lymphomas" [NHL]) at the next conference in Vienna, Austria (see p. 10). Another occasion was the meeting of the Japanese and American lymphoma groups in **Nagoya, Japan** two months later (7-12 November 1971), to which I was invited at the request of Akazaki [23]. At this meeting Lukes presented preliminary results of studies using a camera lucida that he had performed with R. D. Collins. With the aid of this device they were able to sketch the nuclei of tumour cells. They found cells that, in their opinion, essentially corresponded to the cells called "germinoblasts" and "germinocytes". Lukes and Collins used the terms "noncleaved follicular-center cell" and "cleaved follicular-center cell", depending on the shape of the nuclei (round or cleaved, respectively).

At the meeting in Nagoya M. Kojima identified himself with our concept of follicular lymphoma, one reason being that he had found desmosomes by electron microscopy in most cases. H. R. Niedorf had made the same observation in 1969 [24]. Dorfman of the American group defended Rappaport's concept, because there was no convincing proof that follicular lymphoma cells were derived from germinal centre cells. Berard said that this would need further study; later he confirmed our concept.

During the discussion following Akazaki's (Fig. 3) lecture on reticulosarcoma in Japan, I reported that H. Stein of the Institute of Pathology in Kiel had found an increase in IgM in four cases that had been diagnosed as reticulosarcoma. These cases should therefore be considered to be immunoblastic lymphomas. Parallel electron microscopic investigations in Kiel by E. Kaiserling and H. K. Müller-Hermelink had revealed that there were apparently three types of so-called reticulosarcoma: (1) with abundant rough endoplasmic reticulum, (2) with sparse rough endoplasmic reticulum and abundant polysomes and (3) with no rough endoplasmic reticulum and few polysomes. The first type, at least, seemed to be interpretable as immunoblastic lymphoma.

Dorfman presented a new entity that he named after the first patient observed with the disease. Co-workers of J. Rosai apparently described the

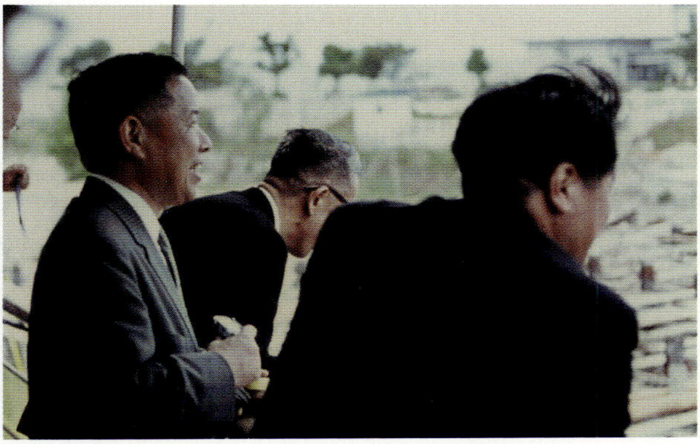

Fig. 3 K. Akazaki, the Japanese initiator of the Japanese-American lymphoma conferences (Otsu, Japan, 1964)

same cases as "malignant histiocytosis with cutaneous involvement and eosinophilia" [25]. The participants at the meeting were asked whether they had seen this entity. Both Lukes and myself answered that we had observed some cases. Lukes called it "immunoblastic lymphadenopathy" and I used the term "lymphogranulomatosis X" [26,27]. Later the term "angioimmunoblastic lymphadenopathy" proposed by G. Frizzera [28] came into widespread use. Then in 1979 a research group in Tokyo introduced the term "immunoblastic lymphadenopathy-like T-cell lymphoma" and assumed that it was a type of malignant lymphoma instead of an unusual immune reaction [29].

During the early seventies pathologists were becoming more aware of some results of experimental immunologic research. Two findings were significant. First, earlier fundamental studies of lymphocyte cultures by P. C. Nowell [30] led to the observation that small lymphocytes could transform into large basophilic cells showing very active mitotic division ("immunoblasts"). Decades earlier Maximow had already postulated the transformation of lymphocytes and had used the terms "micro-", "meso-" and "macrolymphocytes". Second, two functionally different lymphocyte systems were discovered, namely, the B- and T-lymphocyte systems. The topography, morphology and function of these systems were investigated with great intensity. Both discoveries challenged me and others to investigate whether the morphological variants of malignant lymphoma are in fact different expressions of the various types of lymphocytes and their derivatives. We were encouraged by F. J. Keuning and his research group in Groningen, The Netherlands. He and his co-workers visited the Institute of Pathology in

Kiel and he also found a specialized immunochemist (H. Bouman) to work with us.

Hence results of experimental immunologic research were the impulse for lymphoma studies by a research group in Los Angeles, CA (USA; Lukes and co-workers) and by the research group in Kiel. Both groups began their work at about the same time in 1971. Lukes was assisted by Collins in cytological studies using a camera lucida, on which he based his first publications (see p. 8). In Kiel fortunate circumstances made it possible for Stein to do immunochemical analyses of lymphoma tissue homogenates. M. R. Parwaresch provided the technical know-how of his laboratory. Just at the right moment during the routine diagnosis of lymph node biopsies we noticed several large-cell lymphomas that were so strongly basophilic that there was good reason to suspect increased production of proteins in the tumour cells. Further analysis revealed that the tumour cells actually contained large amounts of IgM [31]. This encouraged us to look for increases in IgM and other types of immunoglobulin (Ig) in other types of lymphoma. The search was successful.

At the 2nd International Workshop on Chemo- and Immunotherapy of Leukaemia and Malignant Lymphomas in **Vienna** in 1972 (20 March) surprisingly little international attention was paid to the presentations given by myself and Stein [32]. We reported on the first 27 cases of malignant lymphoma (including plasmacytoma) that had been investigated with immunochemical methods. Consequences could be drawn from the results of these studies, together with the morphology of the tumours, indicating that the classification of lymphomas should be revised. In 11 of the 27 cases of malignant lymphoma the tissue contained increased amounts of IgM, but only some of these cases also showed paraproteinaemia. Up to this time most of the cases would have been diagnosed as reticulosarcoma. There were also some tumours, however, that displayed histologically a monotonous-looking increase in lymphocytes together with plasmacytoid cells; we used the term "immunocytoma" for such cases. The most important diagnostic criterion was found in these cases with periodic acid-Schiff (PAS) staining: "intranuclear" globular inclusions, which are known as Dutcher bodies in Waldenström's macroglobulinaemia. Since paraproteins could not be found in the blood in a few of these cases, we concluded that there are cases of immunocytoma without paraproteinaemia, i.e. Waldenström's macroglobulinaemia without paraproteinaemia. This phenomenon had already been published in 1971 by J. Diebold et al. [33] and was described in detail by Kaiserling et al. [34]. In all future histological analyses we therefore included PAS staining in order to make Ig retained in the tumour cells visible.

The results of these investigations were the beginning of the path toward a biological understanding of malignant lymphomas. At the time the differentiation of B- and T-cell lymphomas was still an unmet challenge, as proposed by R. A. Good as early as 1965 [35].

2.4 THE KIEL LYMPHOMA STUDY GROUP

The meeting in Vienna was hosted by Stacher (Fig. 4), who thereby opened the door previously held closed by clinicians. Directly after our presentations a group of Austrian and German clinicians got together and agreed to send specially prepared material from all of their suspected cases of malignant lymphoma to Kiel. This group later became known as the "Kiel Lymphoma Study Group". One Austrian and eight German hospitals were represented in the group.[1] In September 1972 G. Brittinger (Fig. 5) of Essen, Germany took over as head of the group. All of the participating clinicians were required to send the following material from each case: a fresh biopsy specimen, tissue fixed in formaldehyde (intended for embedding in paraffin) and tissue fixed in glutaraldehyde (for electron microscopy). They also agreed to prepare 10 imprints of tumour tissue (for Pappenheim and histochemical stainings), 10 blood smears (to be stained by the same methods as the imprints) and 10 ml serum (for Ig analysis). Finally, they had to fill out a detailed questionnaire with all the relevant clinical data.

The clinicians' willingness to participate made a multiparameter study possible for the first time. In the laboratories in Kiel biopsies from all suspected cases of malignant lymphoma were embedded in paraffin by an optimized method. Sections were stained with Giemsa and these were compared with Pappenheim-stained imprints. Sections were also stained with H&E, PAS, and the silver impregnation technique (Gomori). Imprints were analyzed by cytochemistry (enzyme cytochemistry) in the laboratory of Leder. The electron microscopic analyses were performed by Kaiserling. Tissue

1 The Austrian clinician was A. Stacher (Vienna). The German clinicians were H. Bartels (Lübeck); Irene Boll (Berlin); H. Begemann and co-workers W. Kaboth, P. Schlick and H. Theml (Munich); U. Gunzer (Würzburg); K. Mainzer and K. A. Müller (Mainz); P. G. Scheurlen and H. W. Pees (Homburg/Saar); W. Pribilla, H. H. Fülle and U. Rühl (Berlin-Moabit); F. C. Wendt (Essen). A short time later G. Brittinger and his co-workers W. Augener, K. Bremer and P. Meusers (Essen) joined the group.

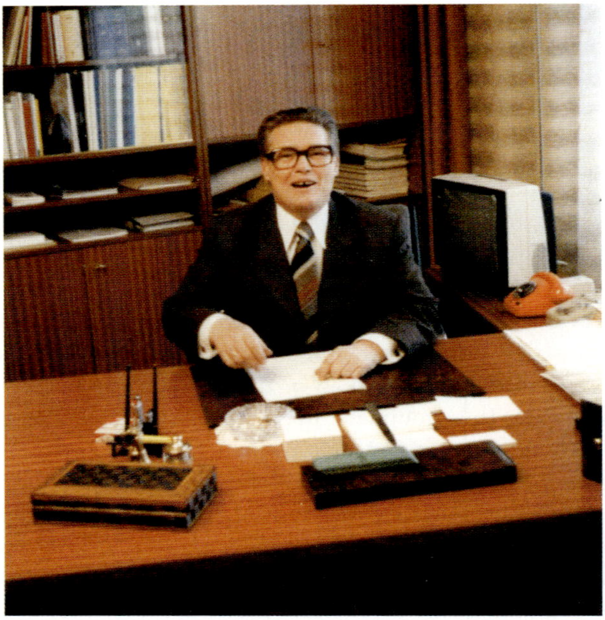

Fig. 4 A. Stacher, initiator of the Kiel Lymphoma Study Group (1972)

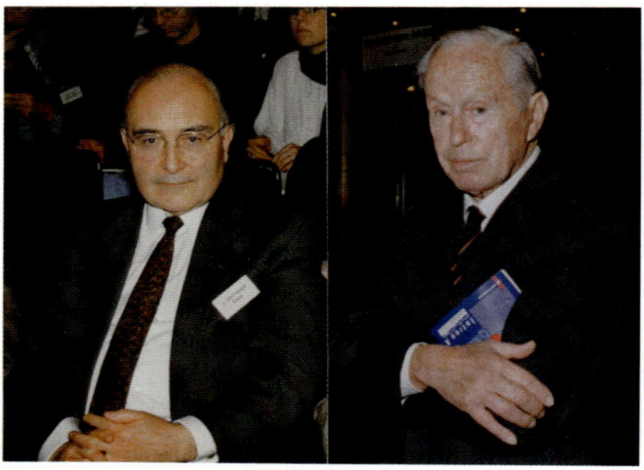

Fig. 5 Two of the leading clinicians of the Kiel Lymphoma Study Group. *Left*: G. Brittinger (head of the Group). *Right*: K. Musshoff (1996)

homogenates underwent immunochemical analysis with discontinuous polyacrylamide electrophoresis in the laboratory of STEIN; later he used other immunocytochemical methods. Immunochemical analyses of fresh tissue were also performed at the Institute of Biochemistry in Kiel (Head: B. HAVSTEEN) by BOUMAN and others.

The Kiel Lymphoma Study Group met again in Kiel in 1973 (1 December) and then in Vienna in 1974 (24 March) to finalize the strategy for the study. An experienced radiologist, K. MUSSHOFF (Fig. 5) of Freiburg, Germany, regularly joined further meetings as a knowledgeable consultant.

Within a relatively short period of time it was possible to investigate an unusually large amount of material with all available methods and to include both scientific and clinical parameters. This was exemplary clinical-pathological cooperation! The study, known as the Lymphoma Programme, was retrospective at first and the results were published in 1977 [36,37]. It was followed by a comprehensive prospective study [38].

Both studies would not have been feasible without the cooperation of the local pathologists[2] at each hospital nor without the financial support from the *Deutsche Forschungsgemeinschaft* (DFG; German Research Foundation) and the *Kind-Philipp-Stiftung*. The working conditions in Kiel were particularly good because a *"Sonderforschungsbereich"* (special research area) was founded in 1973 with funds from the DFG to support research on the lymphatic system and experimental transplantation. The results were appraised on a regular basis and funds continued to flow until 1987. Cooperation between the Institute of Pathology and the Department of Immunology under W. MÜLLER-RUCHHOLTZ was particularly fruitful, as were regular colloquia with immunologists from other institutions both in Germany and in other countries. This exemplary symbiosis of morphologists and experimental immunologists was crucial for the success of the programme.

2 These included ALEXANDRA PIRINGER-KUCHINKA, W. ALTMANN, H. BREDT, A. GROPP, E. LANGER and W. MÜLLER.

2.5 1972–1973

At several national and international meetings after the workshop in Vienna in 1972 the Kiel research group reported stimulating details of the research being done in Kiel, especially by STEIN.

The first publication entitled "Malignant Lymphomas of B-Cell Type" appeared in »Lancet« in October 1972 [39]. The results of Ig analyses of tissue homogenates from various types of NHL, including multiple myeloma, were reported. B-cell lymphoma tissue contained increased amounts of Ig, in most cases IgM. It could be shown that so-called reticulosarcoma was of lymphatic nature (previously and later we used the term "immunoblastic sarcoma" or "immunoblastic lymphoma").

In 1973 (26–30 May) I was invited by A. LLOMBART-BOSCH to a meeting of the *Sociedad Española de Anatomia Patológica* in **Murcia**, Spain to give a lecture on follicular lymphoma. At a round-table discussion I drew a simplified B- and T-cell scheme on the blackboard for the first time in public. This initiated a lively discussion and was the impulse for further cooperation with Spanish colleagues. The scheme was published in 1975 in the proceedings of the meeting of the *Deutsche Gesellschaft für Hämatologie* (German Society for Haematology; see p. 27) and then in many other publications with gradual improvements.

2.6 PRELUDE TO EUROPEAN COOPERATION, 1973

The new, morphologically and functionally based attempts to redefine NHL made by LUKES and COLLINS and by the research group in Kiel stood out against the WHO classification favoured by MATHÉ and RAPPAPORT. A "meeting on the classification of lymphomas" was proposed to reach an agreement, which would be presented later at a lymphoma symposium in London, UK. RAPPAPORT was asked to organize the meeting in **Chicago**. He invited lymphoma experts from Europe (including M.H. BENNETT, N. CHELLOUL, G. FARRER-BROWN, GÉRARD-MARCHANT, IRIS HAMLIN, KRISTIN HENRY, F. RILKE, A.G. STANSFELD, A.E. STUART and J.A.M. VAN UNNIK) and from the USA (including BERARD, J. BUTLER, L.W. COPPLESON, DORFMAN, LUKES, J. REBUCK, L.B. THOMAS and RAPPAPORT's co-workers ZELMA MOLNAR and DAINA VARIAKOJIS) to Chicago in 1973 (25–29 June). RAPPAPORT did not invite me until a month before the meeting. He asked me to send him the classification used in Kiel and slides from 25 cases of lymphoma.

At the meeting in Chicago the participants examined and diagnosed 100 out of 145 cases of lymphoma that had been submitted. All of the other participants had sent sections stained with H&E; only the sections from Kiel had been stained with Giemsa. The diagnoses were recorded in Chicago and were to be evaluated by COPPLESON. The diagnoses of the other 45 cases were sent to RAPPAPORT after the meeting. They were made using various classifications that had been proposed or were already in use.

In 36 cases I was not able to make a reliable diagnosis on the H&E-stained slides. I was given unstained sections from these cases and had them stained in Kiel with Giemsa, PAS, and Gomori. In nine cases I was able to confirm the diagnosis I had suspected in Chicago. The diagnosis became clear in 20 cases, whereas seven cases remained unclear.

Several "formal presentations" were also given at the meeting in Chicago. DORFMAN gave a general review of the classification of NHL. G. D. LEVINE spoke about the ultrastructure of nodular lymphomas. ELAINE S. JAFFE reported on EAC receptors on lymphoma cells. LUKES demonstrated NHL that did not fit in the conventional classifications. I presented the recent findings of the research group in Kiel (which were published later in a paper presented at the lymphoma conference in London [40]). The presentation was applauded loudly, which RAPPAPORT attributed to my good English, while others appreciated the significance of our findings.

The meeting came to a close without an agreement on a proposal for the symposium in London. There was no final discussion of the classifications. RAPPAPORT should be commended, however, for chairing the meeting in an excellent manner; he kept everything running smoothly, he was fair and he had a good sense of humour.

Later that year (27-29 August 1973) I attended the 2nd Meeting of the European and African Division of the International Society of Haematology in **Prague**, Czechoslovakia. F. HEŘMANSKÝ, the scientific secretary of the Division, invited me to give a 30-minute lecture on our new concept in the Plenary Session on the first day of the meeting, following presentations by J. BERNARD and GALTON. HEŘMANSKÝ had heard about the concept at a meeting of eastern European pathologists in Vienna. The title of the lecture co-authored by STEIN, KAISERLING and myself was "New Criteria for the Classification of Malignant Lymphomas" [41]. It was received with great interest.

In October 1973 BERARD and his wife came to Kiel to visit, to see the institute, and for discussions. The BERARDS joined me on the aeroplane to London. During the flight I showed him the paper I was planning to present there, and he fully agreed with it.

As mentioned above, the goal of the symposium on NHL in **London** (8–12 October 1973 [42]) was to agree on a new classification that would then be used by everyone. The participants included the lymphoma panel that had met in Chicago and numerous clinicians. RAPPAPORT opened the first session on the histopathology of NHL and, unexpectedly, reported on the results of the meeting in Chicago. He concentrated on the diagnoses made by LUKES and myself and tried to show that there were contradictions. The two of us were quite perplexed, because we knew nothing about the data he presented. Then LUKES [43] and I [40] gave our lectures.

LUKES presented a table (Table 1) comparing the Lukes-Collins classification with mine, which we had agreed upon beforehand, both classifications being based on an immunological definition of the tumour cells. During the discussion following LUKES' lecture D. H. WRIGHT projected transparencies taken of various cells in smears and challenged me to name the cells according to my definition. At the time WRIGHT apparently was not yet on our side.

A round table discussion took place in the afternoon after the lectures. All of the opponents were invited to the stage. The comments on my presentation included "all nonsense". BERARD summarized the discussion by saying that the time had not yet come for a definitive classification. RILKE said

LENNERT		LUKES and COLLINS
Malignant Lymphomas		Malignant Lymphomas
	I. Undefined (not B nor T)	
	II. B - Cell (Lymphocytic) Types	
1. CLL		1. small lymphocytic type (CLL)
2. Immunocytoma, lympho - plasmocytoid		2. plasmocytoid lymphocytic
3. Germinal Center Cell Tumors		3. Follicle Center Cell (FCC) Tumors follicular, follicular & diffuse, diffuse, sclerotic
a. Germinocytoma (gc) diffuse b. Germinoblastoma (gc + gbl) follicular, follicular & diffuse, diffuse, sclerotic	↔	a. cleaved FCC 1. small 2. small & large
c. Germinoblastic Sarcoma (gbl) usually diffuse ?~ Paraleukoblastic (Lymphoblastic B) Sarcoma incl. BURKITT's	↔	b. non - cleaved FCC 1. small (BURKITT's) 2. large
4. Immunoblastic Sarcoma, B - cell type		4. Immunoblastic Sarcoma, B - cell type
	III. T - Cell (Lymphocytic) Types	
1. Mycosis fungoides (including SÉZARY - syndrome)		1. Mycosis fungoides (including SÉZARY - syndrome)
2. ? Lymphoblastic Sarcoma, T - cell type		2. Convoluted lymphocyte
3. ? Immunoblastic Sarcoma, T - cell type		3. ? Immunoblastic Sarcoma, T - cell type
	IV. Reticulo - histiocytic	
Reticulosarcoma		Histiocytic
	V. Unclassified	

Table 1 Comparison of the immunologically defined entities of the Kiel classification (LENNERT) and the LUKES-COLLINS classification (LUKES and COLLINS), presented in London in 1975 (unpublished)

"Rome was not built in a day." G. Tullinius declared the Rappaport classification dead. Musshoff asked "What now? What should we clinicians do?"

Since I had to leave London early I missed the rest of the symposium. I heard about it through letters from Lukes, Hamlin, Musshoff and other colleagues. At the end of October Lukes wrote me that at the end of the meeting a decision was reached to meet again in three years. Rappaport did not attend the closing session. Mathé, however, was there and he asked Lukes for a table comparing the Lukes-Collins classification with mine. Mathé said that he wanted to include the table in the "Blue Book", but this did not happen. In his letter to me Lukes also emphasized that "the important and key observers [D. W.] Smithers, [H. S] Kaplan, [M.] Tubiana and [M.] Seligmann were with us". J. A. Hansen of the Sloan-Kettering Institute in New York, NY (USA) wrote to me at the request of Good, saying that "Dr. Good has generated a great enthusiasm on his return from the London Symposium." He asked me for a copy of the manuscript of my lecture and of the table comparing the Lukes-Collins classification with mine for a review article. In the letter I received from Musshoff he wrote that (1) the goal should be to reach an agreement between the Lukes-Collins classification and the classification developed in Kiel and (2) cooperative studies should be done with large reputable European hospitals. Musshoff proposed the formation of a study group composed of serveral German hospitals. He did not know that such a study group had already been established (see p. 11).

2.7 THE EUROPEAN LYMPHOMA CLUB (ELC)

A month later (9–11 November 1973) six European lymphoma pathologists met with Lukes in London to become more familiar with the Lukes-Collins classification. I had been invited, but could not attend because of another commitment. The participants were: van Unnik, Gérard-Marchant, Rilke, Stansfeld, Bennett and Hamlin. At the end of November Hamlin told me that the group had listened to Lukes, examined slides and discussed lymphoma problems with him. At the end of the meeting the group decided to establish an "informal club for the study of lymph nodes", which became known as the ELC. The Club was to "consist of those of Europe who were present" plus myself. Van Unnik was to be chairman of the Club and would be sending me a "most cordial invitation". Hamlin expressed how sorry the Club was that I could not join the discussion in London, but how pleased the members were that I had invited them to Kiel.

Addendum: As the years went by, the Club took on a few more members, namely, CHELLOUL, DIEBOLD, Y. KAPANÇI, G. KELÉNYI, OLGA MIODUSZEWSKA (Fig. 6), H. NOËL and C. SUNDSTRÖM. Two members, CHELLOUL and HAMLIN, are since deceased. BENNETT resigned (see p. 23). TU LIAN-YING (aka ANNA TU) of China became an honorary member at the ELC meeting in London in 1983 (see p. 87; Fig. 7).

2.8 THE KIEL CLASSIFICATION, 1974

The first official meeting of the ELC took place in **Kiel** 16-18 May 1974 (Fig. 8). In addition to the seven members of the ELC, two observers were invited from Paris, France (CHELLOUL of Hopital Saint Louis and C. NÉZELOF of Hopital des Enfants Malades Necker). At the request of the ELC the other members of the British lymphoma study group, FARRER-BROWN and HENRY, did not attend because that group was already represented by BENNETT and the total number of participants needed to be kept as small as possible in order to facilitate discussion. The observers from Kiel included MÜLLER-HERMELINK, KAISERLING and STEIN.

At the beginning of the meeting I presented the technique that was fundamental to our studies of haematopathology: a precise cytological analysis of smears (or imprints) and sections using Giemsa staining (equivalent to Pap-

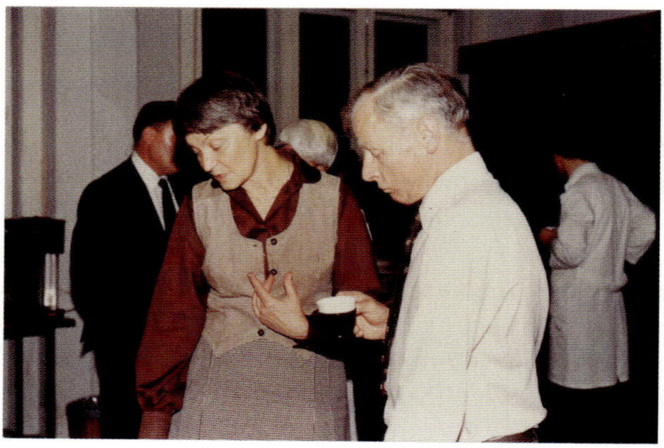

Fig. 6 OLGA MIODUSZEWSKA and A. G. STANSFELD at a meeting of the European Lymphoma Club in Kiel, 1981

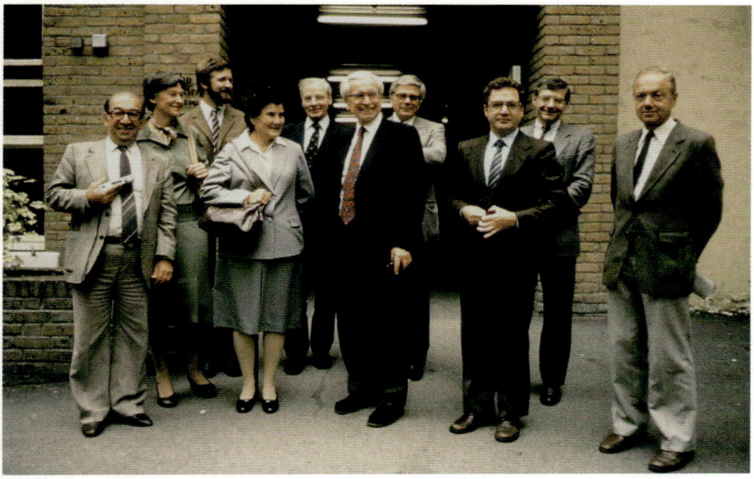

Fig. 7 Meeting of the European Lymphoma Club in London, UK, 1983. *Left to right*: Y. Kapançi, Olga Mioduszewska, C. sundström, Anna Tu, A. G. Stansfeld, the author, F. Rilke, H. Noël, J. Diebold, J. A. M. van Unnik. The other members of the Club (G. Kelényi, D. H. Wright) are not shown

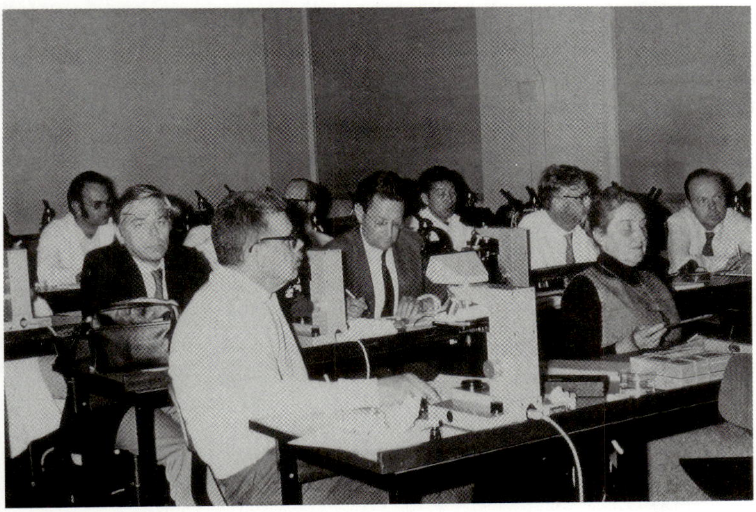

Fig. 8 The first meeting of the European Lymphoma Club in the microscopy room at the Institute of Pathology in Kiel, Germany, 1974. *First row:* R. Gérard-Marchant, Iris Hamlin. *Second row:* F. Rilke, C. Nézelof (guest), M. Bennett, J.A.M. van Unnik. *Background:* Observers from the Institute

penheim staining). I showed my old colour scheme of bone marrow cytology [5] and explained the principle difference in morphology between sections and smears: in sections the nucleus looks like a sphere; in smears the nucleus appears as a flat disc and therefore shows denser chromatin. Then I described the morphology of lymph node cells and how to identify them in sections and smears, paying special attention to the characteristics of germinal centre cells [44]. As examples I used a case of Piringer's lymphadenitis and a case of herpes zoster (with "clusters of lymphoblasts"). At the end I drew the scheme of the T- and B-lymphocyte systems that I had shown in Murcia (see p. 14).

After discussing the morphology of lymph node cells in sections and smears I mentioned briefly the still meagre enzyme histochemical data and showed a few electron micrographs from the laboratory of MÜLLER-HERMELINK and KAISERLING. I did not present the immunochemical findings of STEIN in any detail because the participants were familiar with them from the meetings in Chicago and London (1973).

In my discussions with LUKES he had pointed out that the German nomenclature contained one apparently insurmountable obstacle for Americans, namely, the terms "germinoblast" and "germinocyte" because these might be thrown into the same pot with "germinal cells" of the gonads. At dinner in the evening of the first day of the meeting the other participants told me that I had to come up with two new terms by the next morning. It occurred to me to replace the old terms with "*centro*blast" and "*centro*cyte". Before the morning session I even interrupted the breakfast of H. DILLER, a philologian at the University of Kiel, and asked him whether these terms would be philologically correct. He judged the new terms to be better than the old ones because they are composed solely of Greek forms ("kentron" and "blast" or "cyt"), whereas "germinoblast" and "germinocyte" are combinations of Latin and Greek forms. The members of the ELC were very pleased and they accepted my suggestion immediately. This did not, however, change LUKES' aversion to these terms.

The discussion then turned to the main differences between the Lukes-Collins classification and the one we used in Kiel. (1) The latter includes centrocytic lymphoma (now known as "mantle cell lymphoma") as an entity that is clearly distinguishable from centroblastic-centrocytic lymphoma (now known as "follicular lymphoma"). (2) The terms "cleaved" and "non-cleaved" used by LUKES are too weak for a definition of cells. (3) Large blast cells are always present in chronic lymphocytic leukaemia, whereas they are not found in centrocytic lymphoma. (4) Histological slides stained with PAS occasionally show positive intranuclear inclusions in cases of chronic lymphocytic leukaemia. Such cases are diagnosed as lymphoplasmacytoid or lymphoplasmacytic lymphoma (immunocytoma), which can be with or without paraproteinaemia. (5) The term "convoluted" is unforunate; "gyriform" would be more appropriate. The nuclei of the tumour cells are not always convoluted. Nevertheless, there is no doubt that a lymphoma of "convoluted" type is an entity. On the whole, it was obvious that there was better congruence between the terms used in the two classifications than there was with some diagnoses.

The differences between the Rappaport classification and that used in Kiel were more serious. (1) From a cytological point of view it is not possible to acknowledge that all types of tumour cells can grow in a nodular or diffuse pattern. "Nodular" lymphoma is actually an entity (in Kiel we used the term "follicular" lymphoma). (2) Large basophilic cells are not histiocytes, but rather immunoblasts and belong to the lymphatic system. (3) Evidence of phagocytosis does not always prove that a tumour is histiocytic; the histiocytes could be reactive. (4) The term "differentiation" cannot be applied in cases of lymphoma composed of lymphocytes. The fundamental question is: Are the blast cells seen in chronic lymphocytic leukaemia more or less differentiated than the "-cytes"?

The theoretical discussions were enhanced by examining the slides that each member of the ELC had sent to Kiel beforehand for staining (Giemsa, Gomori and other methods). We also discussed the cases that LUKES had presented in London. It turned out that my diagnoses did not always agree with those of LUKES, even after translation of the terms. In other words, there were differences not only in the nomenclature but also in the actual diagnoses. For example, in five cases that LUKES had diagnosed as "small cleaved lymphocytic diffuse", my diagnosis was immunocytoma in one, germinocytoma in one, chronic lymphocytic leukaemia in one and germinoblastoma in two cases. In six cases LUKES' diagnosis had been "large cleaved lymphocytic", whereas I diagnosed germinoblastoma in five of these and germinocytoma in one. LUKES' 10 cases of "large non-cleaved lymphocytic" included four cases of immunoblastic sarcoma, two of germinoblastoma, two of immunocytoma and two unclassifiable cases. I agreed with LUKES completely, however, in 18 cases of chronic lymphocytic leukaemia, five cases of "convoluted cell type", four cases of "nodular small cleaved" (germinoblastoma) and three cases of Burkitt's lymphoma.

At the end of the discussions we tried to reach a consensus on a classification of NHL. The most important aspects were:

1) We used the term "malignant lymphoma" and avoided "lymphosarcoma".
2) We defined each lymphoma according to cell type and not with respect to the growth pattern.
3) The cytological analysis should be performed with haematological methods (Giemsa) and, if possible, confirmed by cytochemistry and electron microscopy.

4) We distinguished between low-grade and high-grade malignant lymphomas. The names for the low-grade malignant lymphomas ended with the suffix "-cytic" and those for the high-grade malignant lymphomas with "-blastic". This was analogous to the concept of ROBB-SMITH, albeit with different terms. Making a distinction between low-grade and high-grade malignancy was also an attempt at correlation with the clinical course.
5) Leukaemias and lymphomas should be included in one classification, since it is not always possible to make a histological distinction between them (with the exception of chronic lymphocytic leukaemia).
6) Functional parameters should be examined as frequently as possible. This would make it possible to allocate each lymphoma to the B- or T-lymphocyte system.
7) We did not include "reticulosarcoma" in the classification, because we had never seen a case in which the tumour cells fulfilled histochemical criteria of "reticulum cells" (e.g. positive non-specific esterase and acid phosphatase reactions). At the time, only large-cell lymphomas showing an increase in tissue IgM had been found and therefore had to be interpreted as "immunoblastic" lymphomas.
8) We added an "unclassified" category to both the low-grade and the high-grade malignant groups. This made it possible to include cases of malignant lymphoma that could not (e.g. for technical reasons) or could not yet be classified more clearly in accordance with the underlying cell scheme. The classification was thus open for future developments and took diagnostic shortcomings into account.

In the morning of the third day the participants met again to re-evaluate the resolution. Finally, we agreed to call the classification the "Kiel classification" since it had been developed at our ELC meeting in Kiel (analogous to the Rye Classification of Hodgkin's disease). We also decided to come to an agreement with LUKES on a table comparing the two classifications.

A month later (21–22 June 1974) I attended a joint meeting of the *Arbeitsgemeinschaft für Leukämieforschung im Kindesalter* (Study Group for Leukaemia Research in Childhood) and the *Gesellschaft für pädiatrische Onkologie* (Society of Paediatric Oncology) in **Frankfurt am Main**, Germany. There I reported informally on the new classification, which aroused great interest. Thereafter I was invited to every biannual meeting to give a lecture on the latest developments in the pathology of malignant lymphomas. A long-term cooperative study of malignant lymphomas in childhood was also initiated; it was performed under the direction of LANDBECK (Hamburg).

During the three months following the ELC meeting in May the Kiel classification was put to the test in daily routine. Then the ELC was invited by van Unnik to meet in **Amsterdam**, The Netherlands, 5-7 July 1974. Sections from 28 cases were examined and discussed. We focussed on germinocytoma and sclerotic germinoblastoma, which Bennett called "large cleaved". The "convoluted type" had already been characterized as T-lymphoblastic lymphoma.

At the end of the discussion on the second day Stansfeld presented a manuscript describing the Kiel classification. He asked me to read it that evening and make any necessary corrections. While the other participants went to the theatre, I sat in the discussion room and revised the manuscript. The next morning I presented it to the others for final discussion and ratification. At the airport each member of the ELC signed the manuscript, which was to be sent as a "Letter to the Editor" to »Lancet« [45] (Fig. 9). That day, 7 July 1974, became a landmark. Bennett did not wish to be included as one of the authors, out of loyalty to the British lymphoma study group, and he resigned from the ELC after the meeting in Amsterdam.

Our "Letter to the Editor" was published in »Lancet« on 17 August 1974 in the same issue as a classification proposal submitted by the British group (Bennett, Farrer-Brown, Henry and A. M. Jelliffe [46]). At the time we were not familiar with a proposal made by Dorfman [47], which had

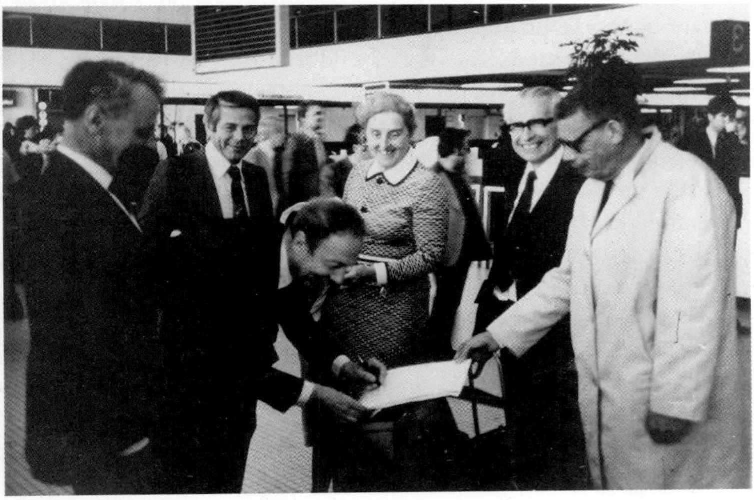

Fig. 9 Members of the European Lymphoma Club at the airport in Amsterdam, the Netherlands, preparing to send a Letter to the Editor of *The Lancet* on 7 July 1974. *Left to right:* A. G. Stansfeld, F. Rilke, J. A. M. van Unnik, Iris Hamlin, the author, R. Gérard-Marchant

also been published as a "Letter to the Editor" in »Lancet«. On the basis of studies using new immunological techniques, DORFMAN swerved away from RAPPAPORT's concept and distinguished follicular lymphomas as *one* group from the many types of diffuse lymphoma. H. E. M. KAY [48] of the Royal Marsden Hospital in London subsequently ridiculed all of the new classification proposals (incuding that of LUKES and COLLINS) on the same »Lancet« platform.

Both LUKES and I were invited to give a slide seminar on malignant lymphomas at the **10th World Congress of the International Academy of Pathology** in **Hamburg** (16–21 September 1974). The seminar was overcrowded; 120 slide series were passed out. RAPPAPORT was there as well, but he stayed silent. LUKES and I presented our new classification concepts and, when we were done, we gave each participant a table comparing the two classifications. The participants responded positively, but many were unsettled and asked for more literature.

Before the congress LUKES and I had had a lengthy conversation in which I asked him to agree to a compromise classification. Unfortunately, he refused, saying that several papers were already in press and that he could no longer change any of his terms. This was a fateful decision. To think how many difficulties we could have avoided if we had boarded the same boat at that moment (!).

After the congress STANSFELD and LUKES met to discuss which of the two classifications should be used by the members of the ELC. I did not participate in that conversation. STANSFELD said that the ELC preferred the Kiel classification. This must have been a disappointment to LUKES. He suggested that another "Letter to the Editor" published in »Lancet« would be a way of reducing general confusion by presenting a comparison of the two classifications. At the meeting in London he had written a short paper that contained a table comparing his classification with the Kiel classification "modified for B- and T-cell systems". The paper was never submitted for publication, however, because the ELC decided that, for the time being, it would be better to use a morphologically defined classification and that there was not yet enough of a basis for correlation with the B- and T-cell systems. This was to be the topic of the next ELC meeting in London (1–3 November 1974). I was not particularly happy with this decision, which was mainly based on the firm viewpoint of GÉRARD-MARCHANT, but I went along with it out of loyalty to the ELC.

A meeting of the **Kiel Lymphoma Study Group** took place in **Kiel** 11–12 September 1974. At this and all subsequent meetings I first presented the pathology of one or two types of malignant lymphoma. Then STEIN explained the immunological findings. Finally the clinical features and treatment were discussed in sessions moderated by BRITTINGER. The meetings usually lasted for two days. There was always plenty of time for discussion and the atmosphere was always friendly. The number of participating clinicians ranged between 30 and 50.

2.9 PRESENTATION OF THE KIEL CLASSIFICATION, 1974–1980

Some of my lectures, seminars and tutorials are mentioned briefly in the following. It is not possible to include a complete list of all the presentations given by other members of the ELC. I would like to mention, however, that DIEBOLD was particularly active in promoting the Kiel classification in French-speaking countries and WRIGHT did the same in Asia. Usually at least one or two of my co-workers were involved in preparing my presentations, either as co-authors or by contributing ideas. STEIN was the most active collaborator. KAISERLING, MÜLLER-HERMELINK (Fig. 10), N. MOHRI, E. W. SCHWARZE, and A. C. FELLER were more or less involved in preparing presentations and contributed a lot of the data. Hence "my" lectures and presentations were the results of joint efforts.

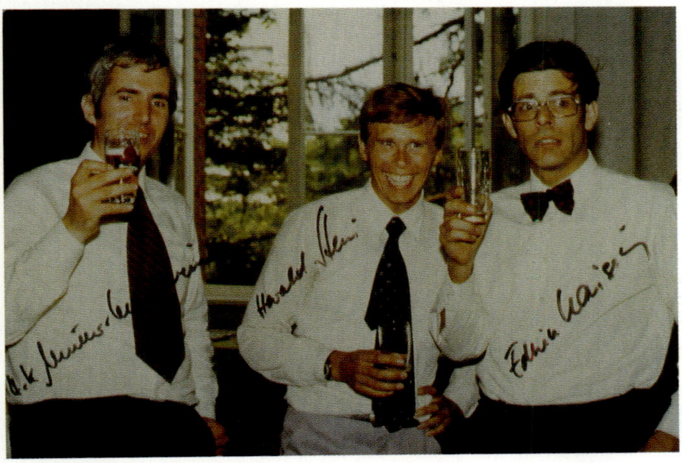

Fig. 10 Co-workers at the Institute of Pathology in Kiel, Germany, who were involved in the lymphoma project, ~1980. *Left to right:* H. K. MÜLLER-HERMELINK, H. STEIN, E. KAISERLING

2.9.1 VIENNA, AUSTRIA, 29–31 AUGUST 1974

The Kiel classification had to pass its first crucial international test at a symposium for neuropathologists on **Malignant Lymphomas of the Nervous System**. K. JELLINGER and F. SEITELBERGER of Vienna and H. M. ZIMMERMAN of Bronx, NY, USA had invited me to give the introductory lecture on "Morphology and Classification of Malignant Lymphomas and So-called Reticuloses" [49], based on my lymph node experience. The participants were surprised, but this was what JELLINGER intended. In collaboration with T. RADASZKIEWICZ he had already studied a large series (68 cases) of primary lymphomas of the central nervous system [50] and had diagnosed them using the provisional terms I had proposed in Vienna in 1972 (see p. 10). They diagnosed immunoblastic sarcoma in 60.3% of the cases, lymphoblastic sarcoma in 17.7% and lymphoplasmacytoid immunocytoma in 13.2%. In 8.8% of the cases they found a transition from immunocytoma to immunoblastic sarcoma. All the lymphomas showed a diffuse growth pattern, none of them were follicular. Numerous macrophages could be found in all of the tumours.

The many other presentations given during the symposium were heterogeneous, but it was apparently possible to draw two conclusions: (1) There is no proof of the existence of reticulosarcoma of the central nervous system; most cases can be interpreted as immunoblastic lymphoma. (2) Microgliomatosis might actually be lymphoplasmacytoid immunocytoma, at least in part. This would explain the occasional finding of unique extracerebral metastasis of this brain tumour.

The presentation of the Kiel classification at this symposium was certainly a shock. I was encouraged, however, by the friendly reaction of ZIMMERMAN during the final discussion. Not surprisingly, the other neuropathologists from the USA showed me the cold shoulder, but this was understandable.

2.9.2 LONDON, UK, 24–28 AUGUST 1975

A brief but comprehensive presentation of the Kiel classification was given at the **Congress of the International Society of Haematology**, two years after the unsatisfactory symposium in the same place. I gave a 45-minute lecture on "The Histopathology of Malignant Lymphoma", co-authored by MOHRI, STEIN and KAISERLING [51]. GALTON and SELIGMANN were chairmen of the session. The lecture was well received and there were no critical comments from either the chairmen or the audience.

2.9.3 BAD NAUHEIM, GERMANY, 29 SEPTEMBER – 1 OCTOBER 1975

One of the most important lectures in Germany was my first presentation to German haematologists. H. Löffler invited the Kiel research group to the annual meeting of the ***Deutsche Gesellschaft für Hämatologie*** (German Society of Haematology). The main topic of the meeting was malignant lymphomas. First, I presented the general principles of the Kiel classification and described the various morphological types of NHL [52]; each lymphoma type was correlated with the simple scheme of the B- and T-cell systems first presented in Murcia (see p. 14). Then Stein [53] reported on the immunological findings and Kaiserling [54] on the ultrastructure of NHL. Stacher, Brittinger, G. Landbeck and others added preliminary clinical findings pertaining to the new classification. The session was chaired by Rappaport and R. Gross. During a spirited discussion Rappaport was confronted by H. Heimpel with the question: "Can you agree to the new Kiel concept?" To the surprise of everyone and to the joy of all of us from Kiel, Rappaport answered with a clear "Yes".

2.9.4 VIENNA, 6–11 OCTOBER AND 14 NOVEMBER 1975

At the **5th Congress of the European Society of Pathology** Nézelof and I were chairmen of a plenary session on the classification of malignant lymphomas. In my introductory lecture I presented the Kiel classification. The lecture hall was overcrowded and the audience's reaction was very positive. Later I received an enthusiastic letter from E. Uehlinger saying that my lecture had been "fantastic". After my lecture Rilke presented the "Correlation of Morphologic to Cell-Kinetic Findings in Non-Hodgkin's Malignant Lymphomas". Further presentations pertaining to the Kiel classification were given by Bennett, Stuart, G. Duhamel and Nézelof. Late the night before Bennett had revised his lecture to conform with the terminology of the Kiel classification, for which I gave him great credit. This plenary session was one of the milestones that made the Kiel classification popular in Europe.

One month later, at a meeting of the **International Society for Chemo- and Immunotherapy** organized by Stacher, I gave another lecture on the Kiel classification. This was followed by a presentation by Brittinger and K. Bremer entitled "Retrospective Study about NHL Except LPL and CLL". The meeting was held to give pathologists and haematologists from Eastern Europe an opportunity to learn more about current scientific developments as well as about NHL.

2.9.5 DAMP, GERMANY, 3–8 NOVEMBER 1975

A **tutorial** organized by the institute in Kiel was held nearby for European pathologists to familiarize them with the diagnosis and differential diagnosis of NHL according to the Kiel classification. At the beginning of the tutorial each participant was given Giemsa-stained sections from 18 cases for personal examination with his or her own microscope (brought along to the tutorial!). During the morning sessions I introduced the participants to the diagnosis of the various types of lymphoma using colour transparencies and microscopic slides displayed by television. In the afternoons further material was presented as part of a quiz for practicing the differential diagnosis of the entities discussed in the morning. The participants were enthusiastic. Several small groups of pathologists got together and decided to cooperate and support each other; they also agreed to cooperate with the Lymph Node Registry in Kiel.

The tutorial was held under the auspices of the German Section of the International Academy of Pathology. Approximately half of the 150 participating pathologists were therefore from Germany. The other half came from other European countries (Austria, Belgium, Denmark, Finland, France, Hungary, Poland, Spain, Switzerland, The Netherlands, UK); most of them could speak German. There were also two paricipants from Japan, and J. C. Machado came from Brazil. I had invited Kaplan and Dorfman to send two pathologists from Stanford University (Stanford, CA, USA); they declined, however, saying that they had too much to do. Presumably, the tutorial was responsible not only for a subsequent increase in the popularity of the Kiel classification but also for stimulating lymphoma research in Europe.

The participants included two French pathologists, Anne Marie Mandard [55] and Christiane Meugé-moraw [56] who were members of two research groups that had independently performed the first studies of the clinical relevance of the Kiel classification.

The Vice President for Europe of the International Academy of Pathology, E. Saxén, reported on the tutorial in »International Pathology«, having attended himself for a couple of days. He wrote that the idea and the organization of the tutorial were excellent.

2.9.6 JERUSALEM, ISRAEL, 17–31 MARCH 1976

Another opportunity to spread the word about the Kiel classification was a 2-week guest professorship at the **Hebrew University Hadassah-Medical School**. I was invited by N. Goldblum, a virologist who had attended a meeting of the Kiel Lymphoma Study Group. He originally intended to cooperate with the Group, but this never came about, even after my stay in Jerusalem.

A. LAUFER was my gracious host at the Institute of Pathology, where I held several lectures, one clinical/pathological conference, several slide seminars and consultations. I also gave a lecture for the Israeli Society for Pathology. After my 2-hour lecture M. SACKS said that the Kiel classification was the only logical concept. During my visit to Israel I had many other scientifically interesting encounters (BRACHA RAMOT, J. M. YOFFEY, A. POLLIACK, P. EFRATI and others).

A short time later four scientists received grants from an Israeli fund to study at the Lymph Node Registry in Kiel for three months.

2.9.7 SPAIN, 23–25 SEPTEMBER 1976 AND 21–22 OCTOBER 1978

At the first joint meeting of the Deutsche Gesellschaft für Pathology and the ***Sociedad Española de Anatomia Patológica*** in **Lloret de Mar** in 1976, I was invited by LLOMBART-BOSCH to give a slide seminar on NHL. The reaction to the Kiel classification was positive.

Two years later a chosen group of Spanish pathologists (80) and clinicians (40) was invited by J. FORTEZA-VILA to a **Symposium** in **La Coruña** with a number of international guests, including ROSAI. I was surprised that LLOMBART-BOSCH knew nothing about it. When I arrived to give my presentation the lecture hall was full. The other speakers were ROSAI, LERNER, WRIGHT, LEVINE, CARMEN RIVAS, H. OLIVA and A. MORAGAS. I spoke for an hour on NHL; then I reported three special cases (monocytic leukaemia, "medium-sized-cell reticulosis" and mycobacterial histiocytosis). The other lectures included one on lymphomas in childhood (LERNER) and another on NHL (MORAGAS).

2.9.8 BOSTON, MA, USA, 15 OCTOBER 1976

At the suggestion of M. STADECKER, J. LONG invited me to **Harvard Medical School at Massachusetts General Hospital** to give a lecture on "Classification of Non-Hodgkin's Lymphomas Based on Modern Immunology" in the morning and a haematopathology slide seminar in the afternoon. Before the lecture I met with clinical haematologists for case discussions. A. AISENBERG was present. I had met him before when I gave a private demonstration of the Kiel classification using colour transparencies at STADECKER's home. During the lively discussion AISENBERG was able to help clarify certain questions, e.g. centroblastic-centrocytic lymphoma with sclerosis, syphilitic lymphadenitis, the differential diagnosis of follicular hyperplasia and follicular lymphoma. The atmosphere was friendly and the participants listened to and accepted what I had to say.

The lecture (40 mins.) was held in the Bigelow Auditorium, the oldest lecture hall at Massachusetts General Hospital. There were old portraits hanging on the walls, primitive wooden benches and an old blackboard. The pointer was much too short and the slide projection was improvised, but at least it worked. There were about 100 people in the audience. Sitting in the first row were the Head of the Department of Pathology, R. T. McCluskey (who spoke German, having spent two years in Heidelberg during the American occupation after WWII), and the "grand old man" B. Castleman. I was cordially introduced by Long and then held my lecture on the Kiel classification. Since I had been told that the formal European style would be inappropriate, I spoke freely. The lecture was heartily applauded and kindled a spirited discussion, which continued through lunchtime. Aisenberg's conclusion was that the Kiel concept was the closest to the truth. In contrast, he had never been able to accept Rappaport's schematic concept, because nature is never so schematic.

For the slide seminar (90 mins.) the Department of Pathology had prepared sections from seven lymph nodes that I had provided from Kiel and made them available to the participants. Twenty people were expected, but the room was overcrowded. Again the atmosphere was very friendly and I was able to induce a lot of laughs. Not all of the participants were experts, so my presentation may have been somewhat above their heads. I demonstrated slides from cases of Piringer's lymphadenitis, Hodgkin's disease with a few clusters of epithelioid cells, Hodgkin's disease with abundant epithelioid cells, immunocytoma of the stomach with PAS-positive intranuclear inclusions, ganglio-neuroblastoma (neuroblastoma "healing by differentiation"), malignant thymoma and Castleman's disease (with "clusters of lymphoblasts" and vascular anomaly). Unfortunately, Castleman left the seminar before the latter case was discussed. In a private conversation he did not agree with me that this lymph node tumour could actually have been a hamartoma. After the seminar discussions continued for another 90 mins.

2.9.9 WASHINGTON, DC, USA, 17–21 OCTOBER 1976

On the way to a meeting of the **International Academy of Pathology** I met Castleman again with his wife at the airport. She told me that her husband had attended my lecture even though he had not felt well (he died a few years later, reportedly of Waldenström's macroglobulinaemia). I had admired and respected CASTLEMAN as a benevolent, wise man ever since I first met him in 1958 at a clinico-pathological conference in Zurich.

The next day I met COLLINS and his wife for the first time. COLLINS and I held a lymphoma seminar at the meeting. Unfortunately, COLLINS did not allow any discussion and consoled the audience by commenting that most lymphomas are follicular and therefore easy to diagnose.

HENRY presented six cases of intestinal lymphoma. She said that all of them were plasmacytomas (!) and there were no immunocytomas. I spoke to her later and asked whether she had seen any lymphocytes. She said that she had found plasma cells only and that macroglobulinaemia was always composed solely of plasma cells and never showed lymphocytes. I disagreed firmly.

Then FARRER-BROWN presented the "new" classification of the British lymphoma study group. It looked very much like the Kiel classification. Could this have been due to BENNETT's membership in the ELC? Later I spoke with STANSFELD, KAPANÇI and S. WIDGREN, who were just as surprised and annoyed as I was.

2.9.10 BRAZIL, 25–29 OCTOBER 1976

MACHADO, Director of the *Instituto Butantan*, organized a tutorial at the ***Instituto Brasiliero de Controle do Cancer*** in **São Paulo**. He had attended the tutorial in Damp a year earlier. At the beginning of the tutorial on 26 October I was surprised to be introduced by TORLONI, who used to be with the WHO in Geneva and now represented the Brazilian government. Since the WHO meeting in Kiel he had been a good friend of mine and he was a critical observer of MATHÉ's maneuver. The President of the Brazilian Cancer Society, J. S. GOES, was also in attendance. The participants were 16 pathologists (including four professors) from different places in Brazil, including IRENE LORAND (originally from Austria), and L. H. ROESCH (originally from Germany). The tutorial was held in a nice room, but unfortunately the Japanese binocular microscopes were of poor quality and the slide projector did not work very well with my colour transparencies. The atmosphere was very congenial.

On the first day I presented low-grade malignant NHL, using colour transparencies and the microscopic slides distributed to the participants. On the second day I demonstrated high-grade malignant NHL, again using colour transparencies and microscopic slides. LORAND closed the tutorial in German.

That evening I attended an elegant reception for about 100 people that was held in my honour. There were many distinguished guests, including the

German consul, presidents of several academic societies, a number of professors and the lymphoma experts. An entertainer was standing in the middle of the hall on a small podium decorated with the colours of the German flag. The consul told me that this was an unusually high honour for me and that he had never seen anything like it before. He and others gave many speeches. I was treated like royalty.

The day after the tutorial M. Jamra took me to visit T. de Brito (neuropathologist), Director of the Institute of Pathology at the University of São Paulo. There I was shown a few cases for histological diagnosis (immunoblastic lymphadenopathy, imprints from basophilic leukaemia). I was told that the University wanted to invite me to come again to help create a lymphoma study group and a lymph node registry. I also learned that the Brazilians had reservations against the USA and wanted to build up a counterweight. They asked me to promote scientific interchange and to suggest colleagues who would be interested. This time, however, Torloni had taken over because the government had provided funding for the tutorial.

The following day Machado accompanied me to Rio de Janeiro to visit the **National Cancer Institute**. I had been invited by the pathologist O. F. de Castro. There the Director of the Institute, A. Eiras Araújo, a gynecologist, introduced me to a full lecture hall. The audience listened kindly to my lecture on lymphomas, but not all of the listeners could understand English. During the discussion there were questions about the Lukes-Collins classification and international developments in lymphoma research.

2.9.11 JAPAN, 2–8 APRIL 1977

On 2 April 1977 I held a lecture on NHL in a small room at the **University of Tokyo**. There were about 30 listeners, including Akazaki (74 years old), Kojima, M. Hanaoka, and T. Shimamine. I noticed that K. Kageyama, S. Iijima, K. Nanba and H. Wakasa were not there. All of my earlier co-workers were present: K. Nagai, Y. Mori, M. Kikuchi, R. Satodate, Y. Tashiro, Mohri, R. Kamiyama and R. Ezumi. There were also a few younger pathologists who actively joined in the discussion and showed much enthusiasm. On the whole the reaction to the lecture was positive. Kojima also asked for consultation on one case.

The next day Satodate accompanied me to **Kyoto**. During the trip he told me that Iijima and Nanba agree with the lymphoma concept of the National Cancer Institute (NCI) in the USA. Wakasa supports Lukes' concept, while Kageyama still uses the Rappaport classification. It was not clear where Kojima and Hanaoka stood.

In Kyoto I attended a **Symposium** on nasopharyngeal carcinoma, 3–6 April, where I gave a presentation on lymph node metastases in cases of nasopharyngeal carcinoma. Lymph nodes often showed tuberculoid lesions and occasionally caseation necrosis as well as epithelioid cell granulomas in these lesions. I also visited HANAOKA at his Institute. He showed me 18 cases of T-cell leukaemia (later classified as "adult T-cell leukaemia/lymphoma" [ATLL] induced by a retrovirus). I agreed with his diagnosis, since the cases were very similar to some cases of chronic lymphocytic leukaemia of T-cell type.

The last day of the Symposium was reserved for discussion groups, including one on pathology, which was dominated by K. SHANMUGARATNAM of Singapore. MICHAUD of Villejuif, France, supported me and the "Lennert staining" (Giemsa). The other participants were L. WEILAND from the Mayo Clinic, Rochester, MN, USA, R. CAMOUN of Tunis, Tunisia, and DAISY SAW of Hong Kong.

During the Symposium I had a chance to spend some time with G. KLEIN and with GERTRUD and W. HENLE. As a 5-year old boy KLEIN saved his own life by jumping from the train on the way from Hungary to a concentration camp. In spite of the hard time he had in Hungary, he did not show any resentment toward me as a German. On the contrary, KLEIN planned to cooperate with the group in Kiel. He asked me whether Epstein-Barr virus- (EBV-) positive and EBV-negative Burkitt's lymphomas differ in appearance; I could not answer this question at the time. HENLE was the person who had suggested that I be invited to Kyoto to supply a "fresh breeze". His grandfather, J. HENLE, was a well known anatomist who had been born in the city where I came from (Fürth, Germany). His father was a surgeon and had been a negotiator for the Red Cross in Japan. HENLE told me that he had been impressed by my photographs. He seemed to me to be a wise, kind old man who was modest but knew that he was very knowledgable. He spoke English with a German accent, so I had no trouble understanding him.

2.9.12 BRUSSELS, BELGIUM, 14 MAY 1977

At a meeting of the **European Organisation for Research on Treatment of Cancer (EORTC)** held at the Department of Immunology, Saint-Pierre University Hospital, I gave a Special Guest Lecture on "Cytological, Cytochemical and Immunological Criteria for the Classification of Lymphomas".

2.9.13 BUCHAREST, RUMANIA, 25–27 MAY 1977

The small Rumanian jet from Vienna to Bucharest was only half full. The passengers were a mixed group of Germans, Asians, one Swede and some Rumanian functionaries. The latter were well dressed and received a special menu with wine, while the rest of us were served a simple meal and beer. The Rumanians were morose and shy, but seemed very sure of themselves. On arrival in Bucharest I had to stand in line for a visa and the compulsory exchange of currency (25 DM per day). I was checked for both weapons and dutiable imports. SORINA LEAHU and her husband, a professor, greeted me at the airport but were not allowed to accompany me to the hotel.

At the ***II. Congres National de Morphologie normala si patologica*** (II. National Congress on Normal and Pathological Morphology) I gave a 1-hour lecture on "Arguments for the New Classification of Malignant Lymphomas". Preceding my presentation F. P. VON GYERGYAY spoke on "The Classification of Malignant Lymphomas". He was very open towards the Kiel classification and even showed my cell scheme. Later I was able to help him move to Germany, where he and his wife established an Institute of Pathology.

After my lecture S. BERÇEANU gave a presentation on the role played by the spleen in the origin and development of lymphomas. Later BERÇEANU spent six months at the Lymph Node Registry in Kiel. He was at least 60 years old and died shortly after returning to Rumania.

DIEBOLD gave two lectures at the meeting. In a conversation with me during one of the breaks he agreed to join the ELC.

All the lectures were simultaneously translated into both English and French. The Rumanian speakers showed colour transparencies of very poor quality. Those from East Germany were somewhat better. It appeared that the Kiel classification was accepted in East Germany and Poland. During the final discussion I mentioned that MATHÉ was perhaps one of only a few who used the WHO Classification.

In the afternoon I joined a tour of the city. The poverty was appalling. The people were obviously devout. In the evening there was a banquet at a restaurant "donated" by Cuba. There DIEBOLD and I were seated on either side of V. D. MÂRZA, President of the Society of Normal and Pathological Morphology. He was wearing a golden medal, was a pathologist and had once been Minister of Health. LEAHU told me that he had ruined Rumanian pathology. His wife was German. He had studied in Paris and was therefore able to converse with DIEBOLD. When it was time to dance he said that he liked to dance only with his wife and daughter. Then he left abruptly.

The next day GYERGYAY took me to the "Babes" Institute to meet J. MORARU. Pictures of President CEAUSESCU were hanging on the walls. MORARU was obviously a functionary. We discussed his experiments and looked at a few slides under the microscope.

During my stay in Bucharest I was graciously escorted by LEAHU and her husband. He was the son of an orthodox priest and told me that about 15–20% of the population are still religious. He was very anti-American. The LEAHUS told me about many of the problems in their very poor, enslaved country, but also about the wonderful National Gallery (three paintings by GRECO, one by REMBRANDT, many old religious paintings). When I left they accompanied me to the airport, where it looked as if there would be a long wait to have my passport checked. Professor LEAHU talked the officers into letting me go through quickly, however. I went home feeling sad about the poor situation in Rumania.

2.9.14 COLD SPRING HARBOR, NY, USA, 7–12 SEPTEMBER 1977

At a workshop on **"Differentiation of Normal and Neoplastic Hematopoietic Cells"** there were a number of interesting lectures (20 mins.), including a few that I had already heard in Villejuif, France (e.g. SELIGMANN, RAPPAPORT). I had an opportunity for good conversations with SELIGMANN and KAPLAN. The latter was very interested in the reticulum cell data of the research group in Kiel (see below). I also met G.A. PANGALIS from Greece, who was working with RAPPAPORT at the time. We discussed his paper on immunocytoma versus chronic lymphocytic leukaemia and we came to opposite conclusions.

On Saturday morning I was chairman of the session and gave a relatively long introduction in which I presented my cell scheme. KAPLAN asked to give his lecture right away and then left the session. D. CATOVSKY, M. F. GREAVES, and RAPPAPORT also left before my presentation. LUKES arrived just in time. SELIGMANN and L. SACHS stayed to listen to my presentation (co-authored by KAISERLING and MÜLLER-HERMELINK) on the four types of reticulum cells [57]. During my presentation the slide projector jammed, which B. D. CLARKSON (New York) suggested be taken care of during a coffee break. He apparently appreciated the work of the research group in Kiel and treated me kindly. The session ended with friendly applause in spite of the problems with the projector.

2.9.15 CHICAGO, IL AND WINSTON-SALEM, NC, USA, 18–22 SEPTEMBER 1977

In Chicago I spent an evening with W. Kirsten, who longed for Germany. He had just discovered a virus in cases of lupus erythematodes. The next morning I visited the Institute of Pathology, where I also met P. Dawson. The following day he took me to visit Janet D. Rowley, an immunologist. We had a friendly conversation in which she expressed interest in having Stein come for training. After lunch I gave a lecture on NHL to about 50 haematologists, pathologists, and cytogeneticists. I spoke freely and mentioned that Maximow, who had been head of the Institute of Anatomy there in Chicago, had been my actual teacher in haematopathology. Afterwards I examined slides together with Variakojis, Dawson, and several haematologists. In the evening I had dinner with several members of the faculty. I learned that some of them were annoyed because Rappaport had taken all of the slides used in his course on haematology with him when he left Chicago.

On 21 September I was met at the airport in Winston-Salem by P. Racz and his wife. At the Baptist Hospital I gave my usual lecture on NHL, which had been announced as the "European Lymphoma Classification". The lecture hall was full and my presentation was received well. The introduction was given by Pritchard, who felt that he was a fellow countryman because his father had come from Nuremberg, Germany, which is near to my home town of Fürth. He was very proud of his German heritage.

In the evening I attended a dinner party at the home of Myrwik, whom I invited to the germinal centre symposium in Damp. One of the topics of conversation was religion in the USA.

The next day there was a gathering in the conference room to discuss cases. The participants were very open to my views, even more than the people in Chicago were, and they were probably going to accept the Kiel classification, since they found the Lukes-Collins classification too complicated.

2.9.16 ROCHESTER, MN, USA, 1–3 OCTOBER 1977

P. M. Banks found out that I was in Minneapolis, MN (NCI study, see p. 54) and asked Frizzera if I could visit the Mayo Clinic. I was very interested and gladly accepted the invitation for the weekend. On Sunday I spent the afternoon in Banks' laboratory, where I also met Li Chin-yang and D. C. Dahlin. The microscopes and microtomes were very simple and old; cryostats were not used.

DAHLIN was the successor to E. HARRISON, who had visited Kiel with his wife in July 1974. It had been a warm-hearted encounter and showed promise for the future. Unfortunately, HARRISON died suddenly, shortly after his return to Rochester. He was highly respected. On 3 October I gave a lecture on NHL to a relatively small group of people in HARRISON's memory. The introductory remarks given by WEILAND were amiable. He cited a few sentences from the electron microscopic atlas (by MORI and myself) and knew about Göttingen (Max Planck Institute) and "famous and romantic" Heidelberg, Germany. My acknowledgement was probably a little too dry, but my lecture was received with hearty applause from very interested listeners. I greeted R. K. WINKELMANN in the audience. After the lecture I was given a tour of the impressive Mayo Clinic.

BANKS was dismayed when I criticized the poor quality of his sections. He was going to make sure that technical improvements were made. He had learned German in school and could read Goethe and Schiller, which he thought was important to understand German culture. He had graduated with honours from Harvard University. He knew and respected BERARD and LONG, but had not yet met LUKES and RAPPAPORT. Although he was very young for his position he was very diligent. His "nightmare" was to find a Sternberg-Reed cell.

DAHLIN had gone to school with KAPLAN. I thought he was kind, modest, and athletic. I asked him how many bone tumours were diagnosed as "unclassified" in his department. He answered that it depended on the type of tissue. In order to diagnose tumours of the cartilage, for example, it was necessary to examine the radiographs, and even then a few cases remained unclassified.

2.9.17 MUNICH, GERMANY, 16–18 JUNE 1978

At the **International Dermatopathology Symposium on Histological Differential Diagnosis of Skin Diseases** I gave a lecture on "Classification of Malignant Lymphomas". I presented tables comparing the original Kiel classification with the Lukes-Collins classification and the Rappaport classification. Then I described the already somewhat modified Kiel classification.

2.9.18 POLAND, 9–12 OCTOBER 1978

SCHNEIBERG had invited COLLINS, J.E. ULTMANN and me to give lectures at a haematology congress in **Katowice**. In the evening before the congress my wife and I joined SCHNEIBERG and ULTMANN and his wife for dinner. I also saw KELÉNYI, K.D. RÜDIGER (of Erfurt, East Germany) and MIODUSZEWSKA. During dinner ULTMANN did not want his wife to speak German with me, but SCHNEIBERG said that there was little Polish resentment toward Germany.

On the first day of the Congress I met L. WOŹNIAK, Director of the Cancer Institute in Lódz, with whom I am still in close contact. ULTMANN gave an elegant lecture on Hodgkin's disease. During conversation at dinner that evening I learned from RÜDIGER that he wanted to organize a symposium with me in Erfurt. He told me that he and KELÉNYI were promoting the Kiel classification in Eastern Europe and that there had been a tutorial in Erfurt for pathologists from East Germany and Poland, which MIODUSZEWSKA and WOŹNIAK had attended.

The next morning I met privately with WOŹNIAK, who said he preferred "chamber conversations" (analagous to chamber music) because it was hard to learn the truth in large groups. The lecture hall was not full for my presentation of the Kiel classification, but the reaction was positive. Then COLLINS gave his lecture on the Lukes-Collins Classification, which corresponded well with my lecture. During the discussion we were able to clarify the differences between the two classifications. Afterwards COLLINS said that he and I should appear together more often (which actually happened). The other presentations included one by KELÉNYI on immunocytoma and a remarkably good one by MIODUSZEWSKA.

That afternoon B. WOŹNIEWICZ took us to Warsaw, where he had established an impressive Institute of Paidopathology at the Children's Hospital, which had been funded with international donations. There we saw J. ZAREMBA, who had spent one month at the Lymph Node Registry in Kiel.

When I got to the Cancer Institute where I was supposed to give a lecture, the Director of the Institute of Pathology, KRUŠ, was there but nothing had been set up for the presentation. The pathologists who were expected from WOŹNIEWICZ's institute did not show up. The only listeners were a few employees of the Cancer Institute and MIODUSZEWSKA. Nevertheless, my presentation was warmly received.

Later MIODUSZEWSKA told me that she had wanted to visit the institute in Kiel but had not been allowed to go to Germany. She did not agree to use the Lukes-Collins classification because she felt that Europeans should not be so dependent on the USA. MIODUSZEWSKA and KELÉNYI each have a lymph node consultation center in their respective countries and cooperate with each other. KELÉNYI's membership in the ELC guarentees the flow of information to Eastern Europe.

2.9.19 THESSALONIKI, GREECE, 16–17 OCTOBER 1978

The Hellenic Cancer Society invited me to give a **Symeonides Memorial Lecture** on "Pathology of Malignant Lymphomas" at the Theagenion Cancer Institute. A. SYMEONIDES' wife and many dignitaries were present. The Institute had been established privately by SYMEONIDES, and he was also one of the founding members of the European Society for Pathology. He had died at the age of 63. The response to my lecture was very positive, and I finished with the Greek saying "I know that I know nothing".

L. BOUTIS of the Cancer Institute was my escort; he could speak German because he had worked for a while in Germany. He told me that C. S. PAPADIMITRIOU, who had come all the way from Athens (500 km) for the lecture, was having the biggest problems. He had worked at the Lymph Node Registry in Kiel in 1976–1977 and was able to come again in 1978 (for a total of almost two years). BOUTIS also informed me that PANGALIS (Athens) still used the Rappaport classification and thought that it would take at least 20 years before the Kiel classification would be clinically acceptable. D. ANAGNOSTOU had worked with LUKES for a year and was now a heamatologist at a lymphoma clinic, but did not see more lymphomas than did other pathologists.

2.9.20 LISBON, PORTUGAL, 27–30 JANUARY 1980

MARIA J. F. DE LACERDA invited me to a congress held in an impressive building built by C. GULBENKIAN. I gave a 1-hour lecture on the Kiel classification, which inspired an animated discussion. The other presentations were given by D. SOARES, FRÉTTAU and J. P. MARIE (Paris). DE LACERDA also gave a lecture on extranodal lymphomas. MARIE was in favour of the Lukes-Collins classification. FRÉTTAU reported on the EORTC study, which was based on the Kiel classification. Before I left DE LACERDA and her husband told me that the Kiel classification would now be used in Portugal.

2.9.21 NEW YORK, NY, USA, 2–8 MARCH 1980

P.H. LIEBERMAN was my very gracious host at the **Memorial Sloan-Kettering Cancer Center**, where he was chairman of a large department. There I met the editor of the American Journal of Surgical Pathology, S. STERNBERG, and his wife, NORMA WOLLNER. She was a pediatrician and evidently an excellent oncologist.

On 6 March I held a lecture on lymphomas in a large auditorium. All of the lymphoma experts from New York (with the exception of Columbia University) were said to be in the audience, including CLARKSON. LIEBERMAN gave a very cordial and respectful introduction. He mentioned my book on lymphadenitis and said it was the best one on the subject. My lecture went well, there was a good rapport with the audience, and the discussion was amiable.

Later MARIA DE SOUSA paid me a visit. She was inspired by my lecture. She told me about her difficulties in the USA, having arrived four years ago after eight years in Scotland working with H. WHITE. Her office space measured only 5 m^2 and the laboratory was very confined. She had to rent a room somewhere else in order to write. She told me that it was difficult for her to maintain her identity in the USA, especially since she was a woman. She did not plan to stay there. Her special field of interest was iron metabolism. She had observed that iron migrated to tumours, which caused anaemia. In Hodgkin's disease she had found siderosis and plasmacytosis at the edge of infiltrates.

During my stay in New York I also visited M. ANDREEFF, an internist who came from Heidelberg. He was doing some interesting flow cytophotometric studies of lymphomas and was able to distinguish low-grade malignant from high-grade malignant lymphomas with this method. He also had news about monoclonal T-cell antibodies, which would make E rosette analyses superfluous.

Unfortunately, I did not spend much time with GOOD because he was about to leave on a trip. There was more time for conversations with the German group (G. STEINMANN, J. BECK and others). LIEBERMAN and STRAUSS also joined us. STRAUSS was very enthusiastic about the handbook and was one of the promoters responsible for inviting me.

When I left I thought that would be my last presentation of the Kiel classification in the USA. LIEBERMAN was inclined to see whether it could be officially used in the USA. That was going to be difficult because of LUKES' great influence. Even though it was getting boring talking about the same thing all the time, I learned a lot in New York and went home with pleasant memories.

2.9.22 PARIS, FRANCE, 15–19 SEPTEMBER 1980

At the meeting of the **International Academy of Pathology** LUKES gave the guest lecture on the results of multiparameter studies of NHL. DIEBOLD and I held a slide seminar on lymph node pathology (including NHL), which was apparently successful. Nézelof (Paris) hosted the meeting perfectly. It was presided over by P. Gedigk (Bonn, Germany).

2.10 OTHER MEANS OF DISSEMINATION OF THE KIEL CLASSIFICATION

2.10.1 ESTABLISHMENT OF RESEARCH CENTRES AND STUDY GROUPS

In some instances the presentation of the Kiel classification sparked the founding of research centres and other formal and informal groups of interested scientists. For example, Diebold and J. Audouin established a centre in Paris, G. Delsol one in Toulouse, France, K. Bürki one in Switzerland, Radaszkiewicz and H. Hanak one in Austria, and J. Jančar one in Slovenia. After my first visits in Spain the Spanish Lymphoma Club was founded by Rivas, M. A. Piris, E. Campo, and others. The tutorial in Damp (1975) led to the formation of the Danish Lymphoma Study Group, in which M. Vetner, G. Pallesen, and others worked together. Some other groups were also established, without my knowing anything or much about them.

2.10.2 MAJOR PUBLICATIONS

On 7 July 1978 **"Malignant Lymphomas Other Than Hodgkin's Disease"** was published. This was the monograph that I had written in collaboration with Kaiserling, Mohri, Müller-Hermelink, and Stein [58]. In this handbook we presented all the important aspects of lymphoma research up to that time. It also included a description of the clinical findings for each type of lymphoma. The book sold very well.

That same year Lukes et al. [59] published a review article in which they maintained that Lukes' research group was the only one that based its work on immunological data. At first this upset the relationship between his group and mine. In a personal conversation between Lukes and myself, however, we were able to reconcile with one another.

In 1981, three years after publication of the handbook, the first edition of the little book entitled **"Histopathology of Non-Hodgkin's Lymphomas (Based on the Kiel Classification)"** (written in collaboration with Stein) was published [60]. It appeared first in German and English, and shortly thereafter in French, Spanish, Italian, and Japanese translations.

STANSFELD [61] also published a precise description of non-Hodgkin's lymphomas according to the Kiel classification. In contrast, NATHWANI [62] was of the opinion that among the classifications up for discussion the Kiel classification was the only one that should be categorically rejected.

2.11 CLINICAL RELEVANCE OF THE KIEL CLASSIFICATION

Very early on it was apparent that there was a positive correlation between some histological findings and certain clinical pictures, including the prognosis. Surprisingly, clinically incompatible findings could be understood through morphological or histochemical analyses. For example, it was possible to identify macroglobulinaemia and differentiate it from chronic lymphocytic leukaemia by demonstrating PAS-positive intranuclear inclusions.

The first review of the clinical data collected by the Kiel Lymphoma Study Group was presented by BRITTINGER [38] in 1974 at a meeting of the German Society of Haematology. It was already obvious that there were correlations between the morphology and the clinical course of NHL.

Data on the clinical course of several entities were also presented at the workshop at Airlie House in 1975 (see p. 47). These showed distinct differences in death rate and survival time between histological types (Fig. 11).

At the **5th Meeting of the International Society of Haematology, European and African Division** in Hamburg (26–31 August 1979) co-workers of BRITTINGER presented the results of an extensive retrospective study by the Kiel Lymphoma Study Group. These revealed the clinical relevance of the pathohistological and immunological findings. It was becoming more and more evident that most of the types distinguished by the Kiel classification were indeed entities. This was most obvious with "centrocytic" lymphoma (now known as "mantle cell lymphoma" [63,64]). The most important publication on clinical findings in NHL classified according to the Kiel classification was a report on the prospective study of 1127 cases done by the Kiel Lymphoma Study Group, which was later published in 1984 [38].

The clinical relevance (and reproducibility) of the Kiel classification was not always confirmed in studies done elsewhere. This was due to the use of inadequate techniques or to poor training of the participating pathologists.

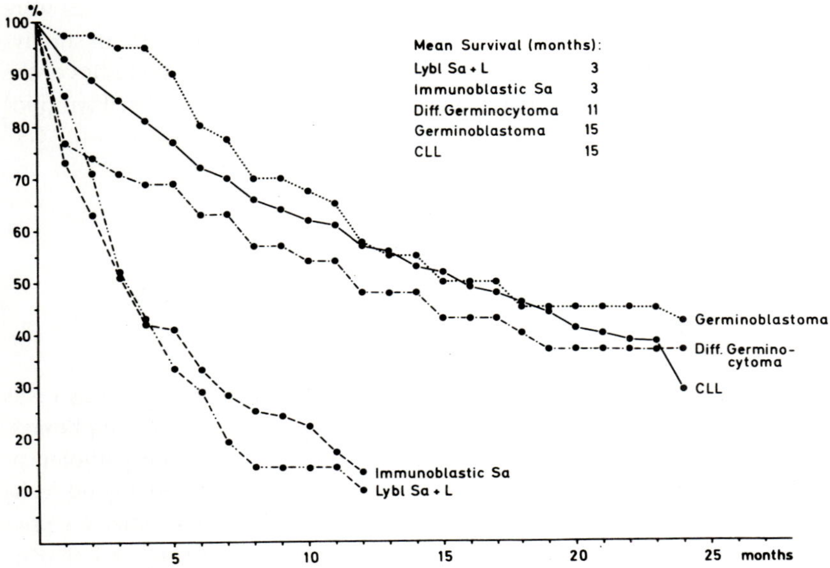

Fig. 11 Actuarial survival curves of the first **retrospective** study by the Kiel Lymphoma Study Group, presented at Airlie House in Warrenton, VA, USA, 1975. Lybl Sa + L = lymphoblastic sarcoma and leukaemia, Sa = sarcoma, Diff. = diffuse, CLL = chronic lymphocytic leukaemia

2.12 GENETIC AND MOLECULAR GENETIC STUDIES

After the founding of the Kiel Lymphoma Study Group fresh tissue from many different types of lymphoma was available for cytogenetic analyses. This made it possible to cooperate with the Institute of Human Genetics at the University of Kiel. The director of the Institute, W. Grote, was an enthusiastic proponent of the cooperative studies. Cytogenetic analyses were first performed in 1981 by his co-worker Elisabeth Gödde-Salz [65] and later by Brigitte Schlegelberger. Both investigators could rely on the experience and kind advice of Lore Zech (Stockholm) and Janet Rowley (Chicago) and regularly exchanged ideas with the morphologists at the Institute of Pathology in Kiel. To our surprise, when the cytogenetic findings were positive they corresponded well to the histological diagnoses. Unfortunately, the laborious examination of the cytogenetic material did not always provide positive results. The data obtained in Kiel were confirmed by several other groups (e.g. [66,67]). Later the time-consuming cytogenetic analyses were replaced by molecular genetic techniques (including fluorescence in situ hybridization [FISH]). In 1985 [68] and 1986 [69] rearrangement studies of the T-cell receptor gene had already made it possible to identify T-cell lymphomas with a high degree of reliability.

2.13 A SIDELINE: GASTROINTESTINAL LYMPHOMAS IN TUNISIA, 11–15 DECEMBER 1978

As part of a foreign aid programme sponsored by the United Nations I was invited to the *Institut Pasteur* in Tunis to study gastrointestinal lymphomas. The institute had approximately 150 employees but only one pathologist, A. CHADLI. He examined about five biopsies per day. He used a good technique that he had learned in Strasbourg, France. In his huge office CHADLI proudly showed me a relatively small photograph of his teacher L. FRÜHLING, which was hanging right next to a large picture of President BOURGIBA. CHADLI's library was very small, but contained a large amount of East German literature (there were no West German or American books). He is an interesting man and I shall say more about him at the end of this section.

On 12 December we started to study all the gastrointestinal lymphomas that had been diagnosed in Tunisia from 1950 to 1969. The material was probably representative because at that time Chadli had been the only pathologist in Tunisia. We sat at a long table with two binocular microscopes (from West Germany). There was also a large photomicroscope and two unused fluorescence microscopes. The sections we examined were mostly of high quality. Although the biopsies had been fixed in Bouin's fixative, it was easy to recognize basophilia and nucleoli were brilliant in the slides stained with a special variant of Giemsa. It was a long day. I enjoyed lunch in Carthage with French and American colleagues.

The next day we worked hard again. CHADLI had some difficulty with the Kiel classification, e.g. with the term "high-grade malignant lymphoma". It was another long day, interrupted by many telephone calls for CHADLI.

On 14 December I found CHADLI wearing elegant clothes (and displaying a Tunisian medal of honour), because he was expecting a distinguished guest, namely the Bulgarian Minister of Health. CHADLI told me later about the visit. The Minister was a convinced communist, but he was not stupid. He was accompanied by eight Bulgarian professors. He understood French, but still used a translator. When CHADLI was asked whether he would go to Eastern Europe he said he would prefer the West and looked to the USA as a model. The Minister asked CHADLI why he did not have an electron microscope. CHADLI's answer was that he did not want the machine until he found someone who wanted to work with it. I noticed that he was not afraid to express his opinions.

That morning we examined some very interesting cases, including one of alpha-chain disease that had been cured. In all there were 102 cases of malignant lymphoma [70], which was apparently common in the gastrointestinal tract. Gastrointestinal lymphoma was three times more frequent in men than in women. The predominance of high-grade malignant lymphomas was striking. There were only 21 cases of low-grade malignant lymphoma, including 15 cases of immunocytoma and four cases of "centrocytic" (mantle cell) lymphoma, three of which occurred in the stomach. I do not remember seeing any case in which a tumour of MALT (mucosa-associated lymphoid tissue) type could be suspected; at most there might have been a lymphoma of this type hidden among the gastric cases of mantle cell lymphoma. The other two cases of low-grade malignant lymphoma were of the follicular (centroblastic-centrocytic) type and had been found in the small intestine. Among the 81 cases of high-grade malignant lymphoma there was one type that attracted attention. The tumours were quite monotonous looking and consisted of medium-sized round cells with a narrow rim of basophilic cytoplasm. Without knowing their immunohistochemical features, I classified the tumour cells as "centroblast-like"; even today I am not sure whether the tumours were B-cell or T-cell lymphomas. Perhaps they were high-grade malignant T-cell lymphomas. There were as many as 47 cases of this type. It was most common in the small intestine. Eight cases were diagnosed as "intermediate" centroblastic-immunoblastic lymphoma. In contrast there was only one case of Burkitt's lymphoma (also in the small intestine). The second most frequent type of high-grade malignant lymphoma was immunoblastic lymphoma (16 cases); in two cases the high-grade malignant lymphoma had developed secondarily to immunocytoma. Lymphoblastic lymphoma was found in eight cases, one of them showing "convoluted" nuclei. In three cases alpha-chain disease was suspected. Unfortunately, it was not possible to perform immunohistochemical analyses.

In the afternoon we examined some other lymph node biopsies (mostly chronic lymphocytic leukaemia and immunocytoma). Then in the evening we had dinner in Medina, the Arabian quarter of Tunis. First we looked at a pile of rubble left over from the prison where BOURGIBA had been incarcerated and that he had had demolished. CHADLI had been the President's physician in ordinary for 10 years (1960–1970) and thought highly of him. He had accompanied BOURGIBA on many trips and had received many medals, including the Order of the Garter, which he proudly showed to me.

On 15 December I left Tunis. CHADLI was waiting at the airport for me with a bag full of dates. We compared our lists of diagnoses and found some incongruity.

CHADLI was born in Tunis in 1925. He had spent five years studying with FRÜHLING in Strasbourg. He was there until 1962, but did not become *professeur agrégé* until he returned to Tunis. He founded the medical faculty in Tunis in 1964 and was the Dean for nine years. At the same time he was Director of the *Institut Pasteur* in Tunis. In order to take on this position he had to pass all the examinations in bacteriology at the *Institut Pasteur* in Paris. He also founded two other faculties outside of Tunis. It appeared to me that he had great political influence. He did not believe in committees, but rather in individual responsibility. This was the way CHADLI acted as Dean and the way BOURGIBA ruled as President of Tunisia. At the time of my visit CHADLI was still teaching pathology at the University in Tunis and immunology at the *Institut Pasteur*. He was a refined but autocratic man and a bright scientist. His French training was noticeable in his manners. He seemed to have a thousand responsibilities and no rest. CHADLI's self-discipline was exemplary and he got up at 5:00 a.m. to dictate his pathological reports.

According to CHADLI, FRÜHLING (born in Florange, Lorraine) had been a kind and very clever man. He had been a professor at the Institute of Pathology in Strasbourg [71]. He had been both a haematologist and a pathologist, the first European haematopathologist to come after MAXIMOW. His death was a huge loss. FRÜHLING died tragically together with his wife when the aeroplane he was travelling on from Budapest crashed in Frankfurt a.M. in 1962. He had been a convinced communist, but CHADLI was sure that he was much too good to have been a revolutionary.

2.14 ATTEMPTS TO AGREE ON A UNIVERSAL CLASSIFICATION OF MALIGNANT LYMPHOMA, 1974–1982

The publication of a whole number of new classifications of malignant lymphoma was unsettling for the clinicians who had felt so secure with the simple and seemingly clinically relevant Rappaport classification, especially in the USA. Now there were several new classifications to choose from. Which classification was closest to the truth? Which classification was the most clinically relevant? The uneasiness increased from day to day. This put both the International Union Against Cancer (UICC) and the NCI into action.

2.14.1 FLORENCE, ITALY, 20–26 OCTOBER 1974

The first attempt to come to an agreement was made at the **11th International Cancer Congress of the UICC**. There I met with LUKES and we attended the session on NHL in which DORFMAN gave a lecture on the classification of lymphomas. DORFMAN proposed a "Working Classification" of NHL, which he had already published [47]. Even though the Kiel classification had just recently been published in »Lancet« [45], it was not mentioned. When I pointed this out there was much laughter among the audience. The Working Classification presented by DORFMAN was largely based on the Rappaport classification and distinguished between follicular (instead of "nodular") and diffuse lymphomas. The latter group included some new entities already found in either the Lukes-Collins classification or the Kiel classification, namely, small lymphocytic with plasmacytoid differentiation, "atypical" small lymphocytic, convoluted cell (thymic), large lymphoid (pyroninophilic), Burkitt's lymphoma, and mycosis fungoides. Then S.A. ROSENBERG presented a paper on the clinical features of NHL and emphasized the high clinical relevance of the Rappaport classification.

During the congress there was also a meeting of 19 clinicians and pathologists who had been specially chosen for a "planned follow-up of the 1973 London meeting on NHL's". KAPLAN both organized and moderated the meeting. The pathologists included DORFMAN, RILKE, GÉRARD-MARCHANT, LUKES and myself. KAPLAN gave a report on the symposium in London and complained that a number of new classifications of NHL had been published since then. He called upon the pathologists and clinicians to come to an agreement "on a method of considering, testing and adopting the best histopathologic classification of the NHL's", with special regard to the well established Rappaport classification. He said that there was no time to lose and another meeting should be held as soon as possible, perhaps in late January 1975 near Washington, DC.

2.14.2 WARRENTON, VA, USA, 4–5 SEPTEMBER 1975

Even though the clinicians were understandably impatient, the next meeting did not take place for almost another year. It was held at **Airlie House**, organized by the NCI, and given the title "Invitational Workshop for the Planning of the Retrospective and Prospective Studies to Delineate Optimal

Classifications of the Non-Hodgkin's Lymphomas". The participants included 15 clinicians, two immunologists, 16 pathologists, and one statistician. Through BERARD I was able to obtain additional invitations for BRITTINGER and GÉRARD-MARCHANT. The original goal of the workshop was to bring the various new classifications into harmony with the Rappaport classification, which was widely used in the USA.

After the usual introductory remarks, each of the recently proposed classifications was described in a 20-minute presentation.

a) LUKES presented the Lukes-Collins classification and added some new insight into the convoluted cell type.
b) In addition to presenting the Kiel classification I reported on preliminary clinical findings from the ongoing studies by MUSSHOFF [72], BRITTINGER (see Fig. 11) and others. The prognostic significance of the Kiel classification was already apparent (Fig. 11). This was not acknowledged by the Americans, however, as later comments by ROSENBERG revealed.
c) MATHÉ presented the WHO classification and added whether the lymphomas were "B+", "T+" or "B and T".
d) BENNETT was the delegate from the British group ("National Lymphoma Investigation"), but emphasized at the beginning that the group's views were heterogeneous and that he could not speak for everyone in the group. He said that only half of the British pathologists actually cooperated with the group and about 75% of the clinicians worked with the old British classification and not with the Rappaport classification. He was grateful to LUKES for the descriptive terms "cleaved" and "noncleaved", but in Kiel he had agreed to the terms "centrocytic" and "centroblastic". The British group had accepted the distinction between "low-grade" and "high-grade" malignant types, but unfortunately still used the term "differentiation". Nevertheless, BENNETT admitted that he agreed with me that the latter term was inappropriate in lymphoma pathology. The British group considered plasmacytoma to be a high-grade malignant lymphoma, did not recognize lymphoplasmacytic lymphoma, and found the Kiel classification much too complex.
e) With his compromise classification (see p. 23) DORFMAN attempted to reconcile the various new classifications with the Rappaport classification. To my surprise, DORFMAN thought that "Lennert's lesion" was quite common and proposed that it should be included in the classification of NHL as "lymphoma with epithelioid cells".

Both DORFMAN and COLLINS emphasized that the frequency of follicular lymphomas versus diffuse lymphomas varies both from institution to institution and from continent to continent. Follicular lymphoma is twice as common in the USA as it is in Europe.

After these presentations SELIGMANN gave a very competent lecture on immunology with respect to the various types of lymphoma. He reported that the demonstration of Ig on the surface or in the cytoplasm of tumour cells is the most dependable proof that they are B cells. He also said that the EBV receptor is specific to B cells. Analyses using E-rosettes and anti-T-cell sera were still causing problems. Monoclonality was not a proof of malignancy. JAFFE then reported on EAC rosettes and surface Ig in numerous cases of lymphoma.

An unusually fierce discussion ensued. Unfortunately, I could not participate in it much because I had developed laryngitis overnight and had lost my voice. The assaults were mostly against LUKES, who was unbending in defending himself. RAPPAPORT and the British group, especially FARRER-BROWN, were particularly angry with me and the group in Kiel.

ROSENBERG appealed to the pathologists to answer 10 questions. In 1968 the Stanford group had already analyzed 400 cases diagnosed according to the Rappaport classification and had published six or seven papers on the results. ROSENBERG found the discussion at Airlie House extremely disappointing. RAPPAPORT said that he was not in favour of the term "centrocytic" and preferred "cleaved lymphocytic". He also rejected "immunocytoma" and the differentiation of low-grade and high-grade malignant lymphomas. LUKES said: "We have to split before we lump." My comments were, first, that we should aim for consistency and not compromise and, second, that surgery instead of homoeopathy would be necessary in the dispute over lymphoma classification. I proposed that we sit at the microscope and reclassify a homogeneous collection. BENNETT agreed: "It is wrong to accept forced compromises." He admitted that he had participated in the development of the Kiel classification.

At the end of the discussion there was a widespread feeling of helplessness. Finally, however, the proposal to perform a joint study of a large collection of cases was accepted. The study would be sponsored by the NCI and its goal would be to evaluate the six classifications (Rappaport, Lukes-Collins, Kiel, Dorfman, British, and WHO) with regard to their clinical relevance (see pp. 52ff.).

KAPLAN was surprisingly open to the concept of the Kiel classification and suggested sending one of the Stanford assistants to Kiel. DORFMAN, however, rejected this suggestion, saying that their department already had too many responsibilities. C. G. SCHMIDT commented that he thought the Kiel classification had made the best impression. He had never before witnessed a German concept being seriously discussed by Americans.

2.14.3 VILLEJUIF, FRANCE, 20–25 JUNE 1977

At an **Immuno-Oncology Week** organized by MATHÉ a large number of experts from Europe and North America met to discuss current results of lymphoma research. These were published in 1978 [73] but there were no reports on the ardent discussions. My presentation of the ongoing studies in Kiel (in collaboration with STEIN [74]) seemed to be more polished than the paper presented by LUKES. A German colleague, V. DIEHL, later complained, however, that I had been unnecessarily harsh at the end of my presentation and that this may have been to my disadvantage.

HENRY presented the British classification, saying that it was meant only as an aid in routine pathology. Her presentation was not convincing, especially because of the poor quality of the photographs.

MATHÉ had somehow found out that the handbook (see p. 41) had gone to press and he had been able to obtain a copy of the proofs, which he laid out on the book table. I asked him about this and he offered to remove the proofs, but I let them stay on display. LUKES had also learned about the book from L. FIORE-DONATI, but he did not appear to be concerned about it. A year earlier LUKES and COLLINS had already been asked to write a fascicle for the Armed Forces Institute, but were still waiting for a final confirmation. I advised LUKES to write his own book and not to wait for the fascicle, which was not published until 1992 (!).

LUKES told me that he had visited Yale University (New Haven, CT, USA) two weeks previously. There ROSENBERG and V.T. DEVITA admitted that the Rappaport classification was obsolete and that there were at least nine types of lymphoma.

MATHÉ invited me and a few others to an elegant dinner, where I enjoyed the company of GOOD and KAPLAN and their wives. I also met the sister of the President of Egypt. On other occasions I was able to chat with RAPPAPORT, who seemed friendly but somewhat distracted.

2.14.4 GENEVA, 1–5 MAY 1978

At a **workshop on malignant lymphomas** organized by the **UICC** the next attempt was made to present a universally acceptable classification [75]. Unfortunately, this goal was not properly transmitted to the participants beforehand.

The workshop was organized by J. F. DELAFRAISNAYE, a Frenchman who had worked for the UICC for about 15 years. During World War II he had spent a short time in a concentration camp in Spain. He was very critical of the terms used in the Kiel classification.

Chairman of the workshop was KAPLAN and the secretary was R. LEVY. The other participants were E.H. COOPER, W. FORD and P.G. SMITH from the UK, KLEIN and K. NILSSON from Sweden, D. METCALF from Australia, ROWLEY from the USA, and SELIGMANN from France. U. VERONESI and ZECH had also been invited, but did not attend.

At the workshop KAPLAN moderated five days of discussion of the various aspects of lymphoid tissue and malignant lymphomas. I was supposed to be responsible for presenting the morphological aspects. Unexpectedly, I was asked to give a lecture for which I was not prepared, since I had brought along only colour transparencies for a presentation on NHL. I would like to note that KAPLAN was very friendly and obliging to me at the dinner on the eve of the workshop. During the workshop he was also a very fair moderator. He said that he would like to accept the Kiel classification, but with more acceptable terms (i.e. not with "centrocytic", "centroblastic" and "immunoblastic"). I was agreeable to this. Other members of the group resisted, however, and felt that an existing and not a modified classification should be chosen for general use. KAPLAN's friendliness and kindness toward me was all the more remarkable as a film on the Holocaust had been shown on American television just a week earlier. Perhaps that was why LEVY seemed to turn away from me.

This was my first personal encounter with METCALF. He did not appear to understand me at first and was annoyed by things I mentioned that were new to him, e.g. the various types of reticulum cells in B-cell and T-cell regions. He became more friendly when I asked him about the relationship between promyelocytes and monocytes.

SELIGMANN was more open toward me. On this occasion he was able to recognize immunocytoma (with or without paraproteinaemia) as an entity, an idea which he had previously rejected vehemently in a discussion with DIEBOLD.

KLEIN was friendly and attentive, as always. The other participants did not seem to take him very seriously. I thought his EBV concept was inventive and well-founded.

The two Englishmen, COOPER and FORD, were also responsive. COOPER was particularly kind and interested in contact with Germany. He thought that Europeans should draw closer together, since we have certain qualities that differ from those of Americans. He suggested cooperative studies, e.g. with BENNETT and co-workers. Evidently, COOPER had been a soldier in Germany after World War II. He knew more about the history of the War than I did and he also knew a lot about the history of German medicine. He was very interested in the data I presented and even incorporated it in his own text.

FORD was a professor of experimental pathology in Manchester, UK, and had previously worked with J.L. GOWANS. FORD was a close friend of I.C.M.

MacLennan, who later told me that Ford died in a tragic accident in Australia. He reported on his interesting studies of the recirculation of lymphocytes.

The third Englishman, Smith, was a nice young statistician from Oxford. He would soon return to Africa.

Rowley gave an excellent presentation of cytogenetic findings in malignant lymphomas. This field of research was still very much in its beginnings.

Nilsson was a brilliant tissue culture specialist from Uppsala, Sweden. He showed me two cases that had been misdiagnosed as malignant lymphoma and I was able to clarify them, but I was not sure what he thought of my opinion.

A few weeks after the workshop I received the collection of manuscripts intended for publication. I was shocked to find that the whole section I had written on histology had been deleted from my manuscript and had been replaced with some insignificant remarks on the lymphoma classifications; all that remained of my paper were the sections on Hodgkin's disease, reticulum cells and, curiously, electron microscopy (written by Kaiserling using the terms of the Kiel classification!). This paralyzed me, just as I had been when Mathé published the WHO classification. Seligmann later encouraged me to complain, just as he had; but I said nothing.

The results of the workshop were published in 1978 as Volume 37 of the UICC Technical Report Series. The book was of little value. There was no list of references and it was not possible to recognize who had said what. The book represented a futile attempt to present a universally acceptable classification and thus an unfortunate waste of time, money, and paper.

2.14.5 THE NCI STUDY, 1975–1980

In December 1975 Berard sent me the NCI proposal (No. NCI-CM-67072) for the study initiated at the meeting at Airlie House (see p. 47). The plan was to study 1,000 cases of lymphoma, which were to come from several different institutions at which the quality of both treatment and documentation were known to be high. I agreed to the plan with just two objections. First, I did not think such a study would be possible without special staining techniques (not only Giemsa, but also PAS etc.). Berard responded that it would be impossible to use special techniques because in many cases only "referred slides" were available and there were no paraffin blocks. Later it turned out that a series of slides stained with H & E, Giemsa, PAS, and Gomori could be prepared in all the cases collected in Milan. The Milanese collection was therefore much more homogeneous that those of the other institutions. Second, the so-called control pathologists were not sufficiently familiar with several of the classifications because these had not yet been published in any great detail. In my opinion it was essential that these pathologists be sent as much information as possible so that they could become versed enough in the use of the various classifications to make reproducible diagnoses. BERARD replied that this would also be impossible and even unnecessary.

The institutions finally chosen for the study were Tufts University, Stanford University, the University of Minnesota, and the National Cancer Institute (*Istituto Nazionale per lo Studio e la Cura dei Tumori*) in Milan. The participants were to travel to each institution to study the case collections there. There were two groups of lymphoma experts (Fig. 12). One group was composed of one proponent for each classification (RAPPAPORT, LUKES, DORFMAN, HENRY, O'CONOR, and myself). The other group were "control pathologists" who were well-known lymphoma experts and were supposed

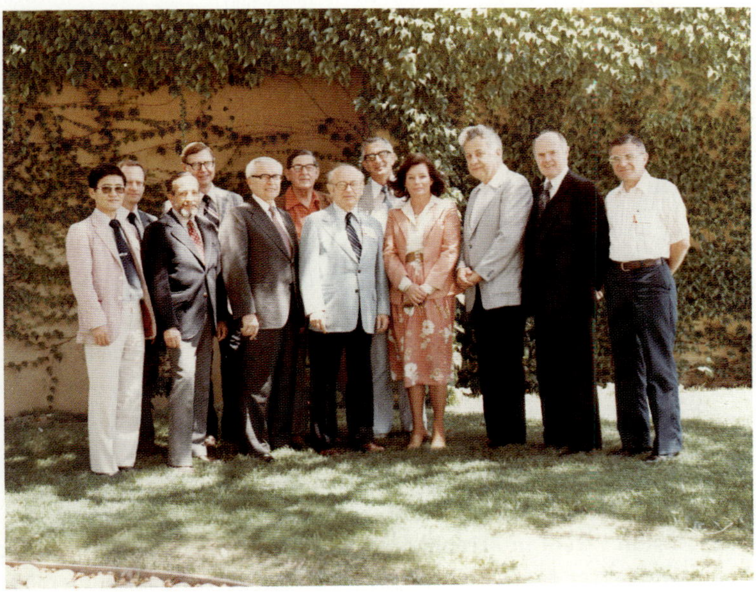

Fig. 12 The six representatives of a lymphoma classification and the six control pathologists (NCI Study). *Left to right:* K. NANBA, G. KRUEGER, R. F. DORFMAN, G. T. O'CONOR, the author, A. H. T. ROBB-SMITH, H. RAPPAPORT, M. SACKS, KRISTIN HENRY, R. J. LUKES, R. HARTSOCK, C. W. BERARD

to test reproducibility by using all six classifications (BERARD, R. HARTSOCK, G. KRUEGER, NANBA, ROBB-SMITH, and SACKS).

The goal of the study was to find the "best" classification based on reproducibility and clinical relevance. The latter was defined only by survival curves, however. The reproducibility of each classification was to be tested by having each respective proponent diagnose 20% of the cases a second time without knowing the first diagnosis he or she had made.

During the meeting of the International Academy of Pathology in Washington, DC in October 1976 (see p. 30) I had dinner with BERARD and his wife. The NCI study was an important topic of our conversation. Unfortunately, BERARD again did not show any concern about the control pathologists' ability to apply the new classifications. For example, I did not think that anyone could use the Kiel classification just on the basis of the London publication (1975) since it did not contain detailed descriptions and illustrations. There was a similar problem with most of the other classifications. BERARD still would not acknowledge this drawback. He said that the study would be done in two years and that would be the end of all animosity and rivalry among the proponents of the various classifications.

BERARD and I also spoke about a haematopathology tutorial held by RAPPAPORT in Geneva the previous summer. My impression was that Europeans were treated as if they came from the Third World; all the instructors were Americans. BERARD said that he would speak with RAPPAPORT and make sure that at future tutorials in Europe half the instructors would be Americans and half would be Europeans.

2.14.5.1 TOUR OF THE INSTITUTIONS INVOLVED IN THE NCI STUDY

In 1977 and 1978 I visited all four institutions to examine the cases collected at each one. First I went to **Tufts University** Medical School in **Boston**, MA, 2–6 and 13–18 September 1977. There I worked in the laboratory of R. A. DELELLIS. R.A. RUDDERS was responsible for the 209 cases collected there. I also gave a lecture on the Kiel classification. In addition I spent an evening with STADECKER, CASTLEMAN, AISENBERG, RUDDERS, and LONG.

From Boston I went to **Minneapolis**, MN, USA. There I studied the collection of ROSAI at the **University of Minnesota** from 22 September to 1 October 1977. FRIZZERA had been responisble for preparting the cases. In Minneapolis I also enjoyed meeting CLARA D. BLOOMFIELD (clinician), KAZIMIERA J. GAJL-PECZALSKA (a pathologist from Poland who had been doing immunohistochemical analyses of SIg in lymphomas since 1972), DOROTHY SUNDBERG (who used to work with the late H. DOWNEY), and R. D. BRUNNING (clinical haematologist).

The final stop on this trip was **Stanford University** in **Stanford**, CA. There I diagnosed 379 cases in six days, 4–14 October 1977. The collection was that of DORFMAN and R.A. WARNKE. I gave a lecture on the Kiel classification, which was received surprisingly well, even though I had been given a chilly introduction by ROSENBERG and LEVINE. At a final meeting with DORFMAN he was very friendly. He thought that an evaluation of the diagnoses of the repeat cases should be omitted from the NCI study because the investigators were exhausted and disinterested by the end of their stay at each institution. He told me that I was the "guinea pig" and that I should tell BERARD about my experiences. Dorfman wrote down my comments, however, and I was sure he would pass them on to BERARD.

Almost a year later I visited the **National Cancer Institute** in **Milan**, 11–25 August 1978, to study the collection of RILKE (who was a member of the ELC). The slides from those cases had all been prepared with the same fixation and staining techniques. SACKS was there from Israel as a "control pathologist". He asked me the same question I had already posed so many times to BERARD and DORFMAN: Why is there so much bitterness in the discussion of lymphomas? SACKS was sorry that the handbook written by the Kiel group [58] had been published so late; he said that it would have been of immense help to him since our previous publications had not been comprehensive enough.

2.14.5.2 EVALUATION OF THE RESULTS OF THE NCI STUDY

The first follow-up meeting of the participants took place in **Stanford**, 14–15 June 1979. ROSENBERG was a skilled and concentrated moderator. The participants included KAPLAN, numerous clinicians, and various observers in addition to the pathologists (six proponents and six experts) who had diagnosed the cases histologically.

In his introduction KAPLAN highly praised the work of the pathologists. This was very different from his tone at the Airlie House meeting. ROSENBERG presented practically all of the tables and survival curves that had been prepared for each of the entities in each of the classifications.

On the second day the clinicians and the pathologists met in separate rooms. The discussions were difficult and there was no agreement on any one classification. Only a few decisions were made. At least the term "nodular" was replaced with "follicular". The term "histiocytic" was also discarded (KAPLAN commented: "Histiocytic lymphoma seems to be a dead horse."). The greatest improvement was, in my mind, the clinicians' coming to realize that the Kiel classification (and the Lukes-Collins classification) is clinically relevant. What was lacking was consensus on terminology (e.g. "cleaved cell" versus "centrocytic"). I proposed a conference of pathologists that could take place in Kiel. Both RAPPAPORT and NANBA agreed that this would be a very good idea. BERARD indicated to me later, however, that no funds would be available for such a conference.

The final follow-up meeting was held in **Palo Alto**, CA, USA, 10–11 January 1980. Unfortunately, I could not participate because I was ill. I asked RILKE to substitute for me. Out of loyalty he flew to the meeting and gave me a report by telephone. He told me that a "Working Formulation" was being proposed for "clinical usage". In the name of the participating pathologists he urged me to agree to the proposal. I was overcome. After much thought I wrote a critical opinion that was included in the comments in the later publication [76]. The participants at the meeting had concluded that it was too early for a universally acceptable classification. The whole world knew, of course, that the Working Formulation was not just intended for clinical usage but would serve as *the* classification of NHL for the near future.

2.14.6 PRESENTATION OF THE WORKING FORMULATION, 1982

After the meeting in Palo Alto the Working Formulation became the focus of discussion in the USA. DEVITA wrote me that he supported it. I answered him in February 1981 and warned against publication of the Working Formulation at that particular time. In my opinion it was created under pressure and much too quickly. Further discussion was of the utmost importance, especially because of the lymphoma entities that had been disregarded in the Working Formulation.

In spite of my protests the Working Formulation was presented during a seminar at the **UICC Cancer Congress** in Seattle, WA, USA, 13–15 September 1982 (see below).

The **second Japanese-American seminar** on the difference in lymphocytic diseases between the USA and Japan was held before the Congress (6–7 September 1982). SUGANO proposed that a conference be held on the Kiel classification and thought that the Japanese concept could be promoted. KOJIMA mitigated. Unfortunately, such a conference never took place. Before the seminar there was also a heated debate with NANBA, who had previously worked with BERARD. NANBA defended the Working Formulation. The only presentation pertaining to the topic of the Congress was that of B. N. NATHWANI, who reported on 62 cases of lymphoma that had been classified as "mixed cell lymphoma" according to the Working Formulation (published later, e.g. [77]). He said that the cases fell into two groups with different clinical features. This meant that they could not have represented one entity. During the Japanese-American seminar I attempted to speak with

BERARD, but he avoided me. I did not want him to be surprised when I defended my opposition to the Working Formulation later during the Congress.

Before the seminar I had an opportunity to meet M. KADIN and his wife who invited me to dinner at their home; MARTHA KADIN was an excellent cook. On 12 September many of the participants went on an outing to Tilliams Village, a Native American village. There I met a colleague from Europe who told me that the 12 groups belonging to the EORTC used the Kiel classification, while the five institutions associated with the USA still used the Rappaport classification.

On 13 September I met with DORFMAN and SACKS to tell them my opinion of the Working Formulation and to ask them for advice. They understood me and told me to go ahead and honestly express my opinion. That afternoon there was a meeting of the participants in the NHL Classification Project sponsored by the NCI. In the invitation ROSENBERG had written that the purpose of the meeting was very important, since decisions had to be made about future responsibility for the project, including analyses of data, publications, financing, and other activities. It was then a great surprise when, at the beginning of the meeting, ROSENBERG announced that he was resigning. He said that there was little interest in the "telephone book of data", but that it would be possible to obtain data on specific projects. Then ROBB-SMITH presented a modified Working Formulation, which was not received positively. ROSENBERG did not want to discuss any of the problems with the Working Formulation. RAPPAPORT was gruff.

After the meeting I met with LUKES and then went with him to the evening seminar. It was entitled "NHL Classification Project: A National Cancer Institute International Study" and lasted for 2½ hours. DEVITA was chairman and I was co-chairman. The auditorium was packed full (approx. 500). DEVITA was in good form, actively participated in the discussions, and occasionally forgot that I was there. The seminar began with four presentations that dealt with the Working Formulation from different points of view. ROSENBERG provided the background. E. GLATSTEIN spoke on the relative value of the six classifications. BERARD presented the Working Formulation and equivalent entities. R. HOPPE reported on clinical correlations. There was much overlapping of information and there were numerous repetitions, so many of the listeners left the auditorium early. These four presentations were followed by one given by STEIN entitled "Future Direction of NHL Classification". He presented the immunohistochemical findings in NHL, beginning with the Ki-67 antibody and ending with Ki-1-positive lymphomas; in the main part of his presentation he spoke about the most significant immunological findings in the most frequent types of lymphoma. In the ensuing discussion a co-worker of S. F. SCHLOSSMAN commented that one should study normal B-cell differentiation before extrapolating to malignant lymphomas. STEIN's answer was that it was not possible to present both normal development and NHL in 20 minutes.

Finally the six "experts" representing the six classifications were asked to present their opinions. I was the first one to speak. I began by commending the NCI for sponsoring such a large study. The study concluded with the Working Formulation, which was just a "formulation". Its sole purpose was supposed to be to make the various classifications comparable with one another. It was not in itself a classification, even though this was often assumed. My objections to the Working Formulation's being used as a classification were based on the following.

First, the Working Formulation was not a system of biological entities, but instead combined entities of heterogeneous nature and separated entities that belonged together. This was its worst fault. Two examples were the "small lymphocytic" and "large cell" types. Good clinicians would soon find out whether the "entities" of the Working Formulation were homogeneous or heterogeneous. NATHWANI had shown just seven days ago that the "mixed cell" group contained two different entities with different prognoses [76]. Since the Working Formulation did not define biological entities it would not be possible to use it as a basis for performing epidemiological studies.

Second, the results of the NCI study were based on an evaluation of H&E stained slides (a histological technique going back to the 19th century) and on clinical survival curves. No special staining techniques (including immunohistochemistry) or other clinical findings were allowed to be taken into consideration.

Third, the Working Formulation could not be learned easily by pathologists because it was not based on a systematic principle.

Fourth, the Working Formulation underestimated the ability of both clinicians and pathologists. In Europe many clinicians were already using the Kiel classification. Why shouldn't it be possible to apply an immunologically defined classification in the USA and elsewhere?

Fifth, just because a classification was immunologically defined did not mean that frozen tissue material had to be examined in all cases. On the contrary, about 80% of lymphomas could be diagnosed on paraffin sections if they were of good quality and stained with Giemsa. Another 10% could be recognized with the PAP technique on paraffin sections. Only about 10% of cases required an immunological analysis of frozen tissue for an exact diagnosis; but even in these cases examination of paraffin sections provided enough information to make a statement giving an indication of the appropriate treatment.

The other experts made the following comments.

RAPPAPORT: "I like the Working Formulation." He thought that it provided a basis for understanding the various classifications. He considered it to be impossible to distinguish B-cell and T-cell lymphomas in paraffin sections. Criticism of the Working Formulation was not justified, since the criticism was based on morphology alone. He said that I was not working in the "real world". He agreed with me, however, that survival data were not the only important clinical criteria.

O'CONOR: An international agreement was necessary. The NCI study had revealed that there were differences in the frequency of the various types of lymphoma. For example, follicular lymphomas were not as common in the Milanese collection as they were in the USA. In any event, the Working Formulation was an improvement over the earlier distinction between lymphosarcoma and reticulosarcoma. O'CONOR did not think that the Working Formulation was necessarily perfect, but that it was "usable and acceptable".

HENRY: The Working Formulation made it possible to compare the data from various institutions. It had created a "common language". Time would tell whether it would be of help in this respect. On the whole, HENRY was positively inclined toward the Working Formulation.

DORFMAN: First he cited KAY's [48] Letter to the Editor in »Lancet« and got the audience to laugh. DORFMAN [47] had proposed a compromise classification in a Letter to the Editor in »Lancet« as well. He said that the workshop at Airlie House (see p. 47) had been very frustrating, because no clinical data had been presented. (*NB:* This was not true, but no one paid any attention to the studies in Germany. See Fig. 11). DORFMAN thought that the Working Formulation was of "tremendous value" and that the NCI study was "unique". He asked what a clinician should do with a diagnosis of "T-zone lymphoma" when all he wants to know is how to treat the patient. DORFMAN felt that my approach was something for the future and not for everyday pathology. He said that he was going to use the Working Formulation together with another "real" classification.

LUKES said that he essentially agreed with me. He thought that STEIN and I had shown where the future will lie. We were looking for biological accuracy in the classification of NHL. There were critical differences in treatment between B-cell and T-cell lymphomas. The Working Formulation was not based on biology. Even though the NCI study was unique, the Formulation would only serve for a transition period. LUKES agreed with me that heterogeneous entities were combined into groups in the Working Formulation, e.g. T-cell and B-cell leukaemia. Biology was totally ignored by the Working Formulation. LUKES criticized the National Institutes of Health (NIH) because the reviewers had rejected a biologically oriented lymphoma research project proposed by his research group. At this point DEVITA intervened and said it was not true. LUKES was also critical of the quality of the slides at the institutions involved in the NCI study; such poor quality was not his "real world". He pointed out that immunohistochemical analyses of frozen sections and PAP staining of paraffin sections are not as difficult as other people had indicated. LUKES concluded by saying that "the future belongs to us!"

The statements by the six experts were followed by a discussion. DEVITA commented that the Working Formulation was a compromise, but it was still reproducible. He said that the "real world" seemed to differ from laboratory to laboratory.

KAPLAN remarked that the situation was now just as awkward as it had been at the Airlie House workshop. He thought that the investigations by STEIN and LUKES were elegant. In Stanford, however, his department received material from all over the world. Most pathologists preferred H & E staining and the sections were often too thick. That was the "real world". Pathologists in the USA were able to distinguish only small-cell and large-cell lymphomas of nodular and diffuse types. There was agreement on the diagnosis in only about 60% of the cases of nodular lymphoma. In the future would just 10 institutions be making diagnoses? He had not seen any study by LUKES or myself that proved the reproducibility of our classifications. Finally, KAPLAN was so annoyed that he left the auditorium. BERARD had already gone earlier.

BLOOMFIELD reported on her own study of lymphomas with immunological techniques. I was not able to understand her, but I later read a published paper showing that the results were similar to those obtained by the research group in Kiel. BLOOMFIELD had used the Working Formulation and a few of the lymphoma types had proved to be heterogeneous.

DEVITA asked ROSENBERG to make a comment. The latter was reluctant, but he said that LUKES and I were constantly creating new entities and terms that were almost impossible for clinicians to comprehend. Clinicians could accept new definitions and terminology only if these were of clinical relevance and understandable. For example, B-cell tumours were quite heterogeneous. None of the six classifications was any better than the others. DEVITA concluded by thanking the 12 pathologists and for all the support from the NCI.

After the meeting ROSENBERG was upset. RAPPAPORT tried to comfort him by saying that the session was a success. The participants from the NIH were also very annoyed. Later STEIN and I met privately with RAPPAPORT and NATHWANI and we had a friendly conversation. Afterwards, in the middle of the night, I had a brief conversation with STEIN, who thought that we should display our colours.

On 14 September I joined LUKES for breakfast. I asked him whether I had been too harsh. He was concerned that the clinicians might not understand that we were actually aware of their problems. I thought it was necessary to poke a finger into the wounds.

That morning I also spoke with some other participants about the previous evening. SACKS said that, "to be honest", he thought my comments were justified and indicated. KADIN said: "You were too mild." He thought that the Working Formulation was of no value. He expressed interest in spending a sabbatical in Kiel.

On the flight home to Germany N. BROCK approached me and encouraged me to "keep fighting".

In retrospect on 15 September I wrote in my diary that the battle had been fought. I knew that the views expressed by the Working Formulation could not be reconciled with the Kiel classification. The future belonged to us. Scientific "truth" would prevail and others will follow. The NCI and the group in Stanford were now obviously enemies of the Kiel group. We would have to ride out the storm. Everything would have been lost if I had remained silent. It was obvious that the Working Formulation was intended as a classification and not just as a "formulation". Many people told me that they did not like the terms used in the Working Formulation (e.g. "cleaved cell"); but why didn't they say anything at the meeting? I was disappointed. At least I had noticed that the opinions in the USA were very heterogeneous.

In December 1982 I received a letter from ROBB-SMITH saying: "I think you are very right to speak out as you did. It seemed to me that apart from your remarks, the whole of the Seattle meeting was a nonsense, but a bad nonsense."

2.15 COMPARISON OF THE LUKES-COLLINS CLASSIFICATION AND THE KIEL CLASSIFICATION

Both the Lukes-Collins classification and the Kiel classification introduced immunological features of the lymphoma cells as an important principle for defining NHL [78]. LUKES and COLLINS based their classification on two new findings. First, lymphocytes are capable of transformation; when they transform they become much larger and capable of mitosis [30]. Second, when LUKES and COLLINS used a camera lucida to draw the nuclei of germinal centre cells and compared these with the nuclei of lymphoma cells they found cells with cleaved nuclei ("cleaved cells") and cells with round nuclei ("noncleaved cells"). These cells were considered to be the same as the centrocytes and centroblasts of the Kiel classification. LUKES and COLLINS thought that these were the most common types of lymphoma cells. Initially,

LUKES and his co-workers did not apply immunological techniques in their own laboratories, but instead extrapolated results from the literature.

A camera lucida was also used in the laboratory where I worked in Frankfurt a. M. to trace various types of lymph node cells. Instead of sections, however, I used imprints and these were stained with Giemsa. This made it possible to recognize the finest of details. For example, the nucleoli of secreting cells (plasma cells, plasmacytoid T-zone cells) were recognizable as reddish violet, whereas those of dividing cells were dark blue. It was also much easier to demonstrate basophilia of the cytoplasm in Giemsa-stained imprints. The results of the these cytological analyses were thus more far-reaching than an evaluation of nuclear shape alone. In Kiel the research groups of STEIN and PARWARESCH also used immunological techniques right from the beginning, no matter how primitive those methods may seem today [31].

The most significant difference between the Lukes-Collins classification and the Kiel classification was the definition in the latter of what we called "centrocytic lymphoma" as an entity, whereas LUKES included this type of lymphoma among the germinal centre cell lymphomas. Today we all agree that it is a separate entity, now known as mantle zone B-cell lymphoma, which shows characteristic immunological and chromosomal anomalies (e.g. cyclin D1-positive nuclei, translocation t(11;14)(q13;q32) [63,64].

In spite of the mentioned differences LUKES and COLLINS and I repeatedly appeared together in public (Fig. 13), since mutuality was more important to us. In the following I shall report on five such occasions.

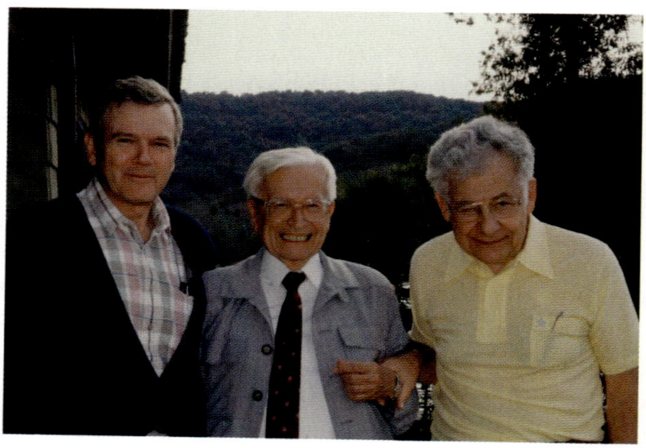

Fig. 13 *Left to right:* R. D. COLLINS, the author and R. J. LUKES in San Diego, CA, USA, 1992

2.15.1 WASHINGTON, DC, 20 OCTOBER 1976

The lymphoma seminar that I held together with Collins at a meeting of the **International Academy of Pathology** (see p. 30) took place without any conflicts. It did not contribute much, however, to the understanding of the two classifications, because there was not enough time and too many entities were presented. The differences between the two classifications were not discussed.

2.15.2 STOCKHOLM, SWEDEN, 29–31 MARCH 1979

P. Biberfeld invited Lukes and myself to a meeting of the Swedish Society of Pathology. We each presented our lymphoma concepts. The rapport between us was good. Lukes said it was possible that my interpretation of the development of germinal centre cells is correct. The meeting was attended by about 100 pathologists, but only some of them seemed to be familiar with the topic. The atmosphere was friendly, but there was not much discussion. In the evening we were invited to a dinner party by Biberfeld and his wife. I enjoyed interesting conversations with Klein and his wife Eva klein, with Astrid Fagraeus, and with B. Johannson (head of the lymphoma division). The latter had reservations against new lymphoma classifications. After the meeting Lukes and I left feeling that we were in complete harmony.

2.15.3 NOORDWIJKERHOUT, THE NETHERLANDS, 3–6 APRIL 1979

The Boerhave Committee for Postgraduate Medical Education at the University of Leyden organized an international tutorial on malignant lymphomas. The programme committee was made up of J. G. van den Tweel (Heerlen, The Netherlands), Lukes, C. R. Taylor (Los Angeles), and myself. Van den Tweel came to Kiel on 6 February 1979 to discuss the programme. The lecturers included J. W. Parker and Taylor of Lukes' research group and Stein, Schwarze, Kaiserling, Noël, and Müller-Hermelink of the research group in Kiel. The other lecturers were Biberfeld, E.J. Hensen, W. Hijmans, M. J. Peckham, Seligmann, Rappaport, D. Y. Mason, van den Tweel, R. E. Ballieux, C. J. L. M. Meijer, W. A. van Vloten, R. Willemze, Rosenberg, H. Kim, P. Lopes-Cardozo, and J. Jansen. There were approx. 350 participants, about 50% clinicians and 50% pathologists. The main topics of the tutorial were the B-cell and T-cell systems, methodology, B-cell neoplasms, immunoblastic proliferations, T-cell neoplasms, and Hodgkin's disease.

This was the first occasion on which LUKES tried to gain a footing in Europe. I was surprised because I thought that we had agreed that he would concentrate on the USA and I would concentrate on Europe.

The presentations by STEIN, SCHWARZE, and MÜLLER-HERMELINK were received well. In one of my presentations I spoke about immunocytoma (including the type without paraproteinaemia). HIJMANS criticized me for not using clinical data when I make this diagnosis. I explained that, as a morphologist, I must make a morphological diagnosis *first* and then ask about the clinical findings. My other presentations on normal histology of lymph nodes, T-cell lymphomas, and germinal centre cell lymphomas were received well, even though the controversy with LUKES could not be solved.

NOËL gave a good lecture on "Lennert's lymphoma". RAPPAPORT and KIM presented similar findings in this type of tumour.

After the session LOPES-CARDOZO tried to appease HIJMANS. LOPES-CARDOZO did not understand his agitation.

TAYLOR told me that he was impressed by the handbook published the previous year and thought it was now the "lymphoma bible". He often cited the work done by the research group in Kiel, used illustrations from the book, and was very fair. He and I fully agreed on the interpretation of Hodgkin's disease.

VAN UNNIK had evaluated the benign lymphomas collected at the Lymph Node Registry in Kiel and was pleased. He told me that the EORTC had practically agreed to use the Kiel classification.

LUKES suggested that he and I write a stern letter to DEVITA and ROSENBERG. I disagreed and thought that an oral discussion would be better. LUKES evidently wanted my help in opposing the NCI study.

The highlight of the tutorial for me was a conversation with ROSENBERG. I intimated that I would be willing to accept any compromises with respect to terminology but none with the entities. I told him that I had suggested a compromise to LUKES in 1974 but without success. ROSENBERG was sympathetic and agreed that all of the problems could already have been solved if there had been a compromise. We also spoke about the NCI study. ROSENBERG thought that I would not be disappointed with the results. I expressed my reservations, which were: (1) At the meeting in Palo Alto in 1980 (see p. 56) there would be too little time for discussion and thus too much pressure. (2) The quality of the slides was poor. This reduced the value of the reproducibility and applicability data. (3) The Rappaport classification had already been modified and was used differently by different people. On this occasion I got to know ROSENBERG as a responsible, compassionate clinician. He said that he intended to support me at the next meeting at Stanford.

2.15.4 ATHENS, GREECE, 6–10 APRIL 1981

The **Second International Lymphoma Conference** was organized by LUKES and his team together with a few colleagues from Athens. Most of the latter had little to do with lymphoma research. Lectures were held by members of the predominant American group, by members of the Kiel research groups (STEIN, BRITTINGER, and myself), by several researchers from the UK (including PECKHAM and ROBB-SMITH), by NÉZELOF, and by ROSENBERG. The conference was held just a few weeks after a large earthquake, but there was little evidence of it.

After brief introductory remarks by ANAGNOSTOU and N. PAPACHARALAMPOUS, LUKES took over and dominated the conference from the very first moment on. He presented his classification and cell scheme relentlessly. Other members of his research group (PARKER and TAYLOR) were loyal to him, even though they may have had different thoughts about his cell scheme.

ALEXANDRA M. LEVINE gave an excellent lecture on immunoblastic lymphoma and T-cell leukaemia; her description of the latter obviously coincided with the subtypes of chronic T-lymphocytic leukaemia defined in the handbook, but apparently without her knowing it. She distinguished two types of T-immunoblastic lymphoma, one of which corresponded to T-zone lymphoma of the Kiel classification. She was a clinician who worked with LUKES.

On the following day STEIN gave a lecture on B-cell differentiation. His techniques and illustrations were of very high quality. Many listeners wished to speak with him afterwards, but unfortunately he had to leave.

The topics of my two lectures were germinal centre cell lymphomas and immuncytoma. The audience was very interested and the Greek listeners thought that my presentations were clear and of significance. A. VIDEBAEK criticized me for finding immunocytoma in too many cases of Sjögren's syndrome (he apparently meant "incidence" instead of "frequency"). LUKES commented that his germinal centre cell scheme (which I considered to be incorrect) was based mainly on the study of lymphomas.

The main topic of the next day's session was immunoblastic proliferation. In his introduction LUKES spoke about immunoblastic lymphadenopathy. NÉZELOF reported on malignant lymphomas in patients with immune deficiency and on histiocytosis X. RILKE presented malignant histiocytosis. R. MAURER gave a talk on thyroid lymphomas; he cited from the American literature, but did not mention the work of SCHWARZE in Kiel.

During the midday break I enjoyed a refreshing conversation with ROBB-SMITH and his wife. She was a haematologist, specializing in the testing of blood groups. She was sympathetic about our classification problems because there were similar arguments over blood groups. ROBB-SMITH agreed with my oral and written opinions of the Working Formulation and was very encouraging.

In the afternoon I had another opportunity to speak with ROSENBERG. I plead with him to at least leave the tables out of his lecture on the Working Formulation. My impression was that he understood my concerns about the consequences of the Working Formulation.

On the fourth day of the conference the topic was T cells. STEIN gave the introductory lecture. No other members of our research group spoke that day. ROBB-SMITH gave a presentation on T-cell lymphomas in the skin, with special emphasis on mycosis fungoides.

A round table discussion was added to the programme, to which RILKE, LUKES, and I were invited to contribute. LUKES asked me about the reproducibility of diagnoses of T-cell lymphomas according to the Kiel classificaton. I responded that VAN UNNIK had studied this specifically and found that the Kiel classification showed the best reproducibility. LUKES thought that these results were "subjective".

In the evening I was invited out by M. PAPAMICHAIL, an internationally known immunologist who had held a good lecture. He was interested in the work of STEIN and tried, unsuccessfully, to find him to ask him for some antibodies. We were joined by ROSENBERG, PANGALIS, and LUKES. PANGALIS wondered why RAPPAPORT had not been invited to the conference. LUKES said that he wanted to avoid a repeat of an unfriendly encounter in Noordwijkerhout.

The focus of the final day of the conference was Hodgkin's disease. LUKES gave the main lecture. Even though I was not prepared, I had to speak about "epithelioid cellular lymphogranulomatosis" ("Lennert's lymphoma"). I mentioned that monoclonal antibodies to Sternberg-Reed cells would be needed to determine whether this type of lymphoma belongs to the NHL or to Hodgkin's disease.

In the afternoon ROSENBERG presented the Working Formulation. He showed an abridged table without subgroups and without a miscellaneous group. This was a clever way to avoid conflict. He said that he was not the inventor of the Working Formulation and that it had been agreed upon by the partipants in the NCI study. He mentioned that I was the one who suffered the most because the Working Formulation did not use terms from the Kiel classification. Everyone should be grateful for the clinical data being made available from the study. ROSENBERG used the survival curves for the Lukes-Collins classification to explain the results. In the discussion LUKES expressed only concern that chronic lymphocytic leukaemia and immunocytoma had been combined in one group and that rare entities were ignored by the Working Formulation. He presented a series of confusing tables and curves; the audience's reaction was reserved but positive. Then I was given the final five minutes of the dicussion to express my views. I said that I was very worried that it would take years to learn the Working Formulation and more years to forget it. The Working Formulation was a step backwards and would delay progress. Terms such as "cleaved cell" were foolish. I was very sad because the Working Formulation was a misfortune. The audience responded with loud applause. Afterwards many listeners (including ROBB-SMITH, MEUGÉ, and many people I did not know) expressed their appreciation to me personally.

LUKES closed the meeting by saying that he would be going to Kiel to clarify the remaining discrepancies between our two concepts. He said that the only problem was the difference in interpretation of germinal centre cell tumours.

After the conference I spent a day with PAPADIMITRIOU in Delphi. We met many "lymphomaniacs" there (this was ROSENBERG's term for lymphoma experts). The next day PAPACHARALAMPOUS invited me to his summer house. He wondered why Germany was still divided and said that Europe needs a strong Germany. He had suffered during the German occupation of Greece in World War II. He said that 80% of the Greeks were anti-American (because of Cyprus). We agreed that there should be a joint meeting of German and Greek pathologists in either Germany or Greece in two years; but this plan was later forgotten.

2.15.5 KIEL, GERMANY, 16–21 APRIL 1981

LUKES kept the promise he had made in Athens and came to Kiel together with COLLINS in order to reconcile the remaining differences between their classification and the Kiel classification. After lengthy discussions, COLLINS and I asked LUKES to draft a joint publication, which LUKES gladly agreed to do. The graphic designer at the institute in Kiel, W. VATER, prepared a schematic drawing demonstrating the "only" but elementary difference between the two classifications: in the Kiel classification centrocytic lymphoma is sharply distinguished from centroblastic-centrocytic lymphoma, whereas LUKES and COLLINS did not agree that centrocytic lymphoma is a separate entity.

At the end of LUKES' and COLLINS' visit we entitled the paper "concordance" of the two classifications and believed, mistakenly, that all the discrepancy problems had been solved. In particular, we thought that it was just a matter of nomenclature and not of definitions [77].

2.16 ACCEPTANCE OF THE KIEL CLASSIFICATION, 1981–1987

In 1981 and the years following a number of important congresses and meetings focussing on malignant lymphomas as a whole took place. Immunology was playing an ever greater role and the Kiel classification was often at the centre of attention. Our classification was presented for discussion not only by our research group, but by other supporters as well. After many presentations in Europe and the USA the discussion spread to South America, China, and Japan. The other members of the ELC also made significant contributions in the form of lectures and seminars in order to spread information about the Kiel classification. On the whole there was great interest in accepting the classification, even though it was not always easy to get used to the new terms. Eventually, however, the terms were accepted, especially since it was soon recognized that the Working Formulation was scientifically untenable. The Lukes-Collins classification, on the other hand, did not receive as much attention because it took so long for the fascicle to be published (by the Armed Forces Institute).

The most important occasions that focussed on the Kiel classification will be described in this section. The next chapters will deal with the final phase of the development of the European Association for Haematopathology out of the European Lymphoma Study Group.

2.16.1 VIENNA, 15–18 FEBRUARY 1981

A large international **Leukaemia Marker Conference** was organized by W. Knapp [79]. The lecturers included many well known experts in the new field of immunomorphology (e.g. Seligmann, Schlossman). Stein gave a brilliant lecture on the immunohistology of B-cell lymphomas. At the end of the conference there was a round table discussion moderated by H. Huber. This finished with an aggressive debate between Schlossman and myself. He had misunderstood me when I said that it was possible to recognize the B-cell or T-cell nature of many lymphomas just by light microscopy (with appropriate techniques) and that a precise morphological analysis was necessary before applying immunological methods. Schlossman thought that I was overestimating morphology and ignoring immunology. I did not succeed in explaining this misunderstanding. The next time we saw each other (at a meeting in Squaw Valley, see p. 75), however, Schlossman tried to make amends by offering me some new antibodies.

During the rest of the round table discussion Seligmann was fair to the research group in Kiel in his argumentation, whereas he was not so kind toward LUKES' group. G. JANOSSY contributed lengthy remarks on acute lymphocytic leukaemia etc.; he showed his support by mentioning my name several times.

There were other interesting encounters at the conference. For example, one of BERARD's co-workers was highly critical of STEIN's presentation of centroblastic-centrocytic lymphoma without an increase in Ig. I. GREEN, on the other hand, apparently had a favourable opinion of STEIN. As for the Working Formulation, J. H. KERSEY said that it represented "regression" and not "progression". He did not think that Europeans would use it. GREAVES apologized for his aggressive answer to my question about the decisive criterion for making an immunological diagnosis.

After the conference I came to the conclusion that the Kiel classification was already being used by many others, with no great stir. The Rappaport classification was hardly mentioned at all and it appeared to have gone out of fashion. The "lymphoma world" had certainly changed!

2.16.2 LJUBLJANA, YUGOSLAVIA, 14–15 APRIL 1981

At the suggestion of RILKE, I was invited by MARIJA US-KRAŠOVEC to hold a seminar on NHL. SCHWARZE was also invited. On the first day I held lectures on normal lymphatic tissue and low-grade malignant NHL. There were about 50 listeners, but hardly any of them understood English. The lecture hall was beautiful; it was located in the hospital where President TITO died.

There were more lectures on the second day, including one by SCHWARZE. The audience was attentive, but had some difficulty with all the new terms and information. I suggested the formation of a lymphoma study group which could send delegates to our workshops. Later JANČAR came to Kiel for three months and stayed in contact after that.

During my visit I had an opportunity to spend time with D. FERLUGA, professor of pathology and vice president of the European Society of Pathology.

The hospitality of US-KRAŠOVEC was overwhelming. She was an enthusiastic cytologist. Unfortunately, she was having problems with her eyes and could no longer use a microscope. The simple cancer institute where she and JANČAR worked was located in old barracks that had been built by Empress MARIA THERESA. The institute had a well functioning cancer registry that collected cases from all over Slovenia.

None of my hosts were communists. Only about 5% of the employees at the institution were, and only those in top positions needed to be members of the Party. I noticed that everyone felt free to speak as they wished.

2.16.3 ERICE, SICILY, 3–9 MAY 1981

The International School of Medical Sciences offered the **"15th Course: Advances in Lymphoproliferative Disorders"** at the Centre for Scientific Culture. There were many distinguished guests, including BERNARD, J. BRETON-GORIUS, and R. C. GALLO. I gave a lecture on "Immunological Aspects and Pathology of NHL".

The atmosphere at the meeting was congenial and the reaction to my presentation was positive. I had an opportunity to meet BRETON-GORIUS and invited her to Kiel and to the congress of the German Society of Pathology in Lucerne (see p. 85). The host, A. CAJOZZO, was very kind to me and arranged an audience with the Bishop of Monreale (near Palermo), who showed me the cathedral.

2.16.4 ERFURT, GERMANY, 13 MAY 1981

After attending a meeting of the *Deutsche Akademie der Naturforscher Leopoldina* (German Academy of Natural Scientists Leopoldina) in Halle, Germany, RÜDIGER accompanied me to Erfurt, where I gave a seminar on NHL for pathologists from East Germany and neighboring Eastern European countries. The participants included MIODUSZEWSKA, H. NIZZE, W. WÖCKEL, and P. STEUDTE. The city of Erfurt was depressing. D. SCHREIBER hosted the seminar and invited me to dinner at his home, where everything was elegant. That evening there were reports on the television of the assault on the Pope, which deeply upset MIODUSZEWSKA. Those guests who were Communists said that nothing like that would ever happen in East Germany and turned off the television. I boldly expressed my Western opinions.

2.16.5 MONTREAL, CANADA, 17–21 SEPTEMBER 1981

Before the congress of the **International Society of Lymphology** I had an opportunity to spend a few days in Montreal. The first people I met were P. BETTEZ and M. TREMBLAY of McGill University. The latter told me some news from Paris, where he had been just recently. Later he came and spent a week in Kiel and he also attended the meeting on the Working Formulation in Seattle, WA (see pp. 57ff.). On Sunday before the congress I met with R. GARNEAU from Quebec. He had trained with C. OBERLING and ROBB-SMITH and had taught in Dijon, France. He was a haematopathologist and now director of a hospital. He was an enthusiastic supporter of the Kiel classification. He gave me a copy of the pathology textbook of which he was co-author [80].

In the afternoon before the congress a slide seminar was held for Canadian pathologists. The cases were submitted by the Quebec Association of Pathologists. Unfortunately, there were problems with the slide projector, so I could not show any of my colour transparencies. The seminar lasted all afternoon and the atmosphere was friendly and relaxed.

That evening I had dinner with Garneau and R. Madarnas. The latter came to Kiel in 1993 and spent six months working with me.

The congress began on 21 September. The president of the Society, R. Belanger, gave an eloquent opening address. Then I was introduced by Madarnas. I gave a lecture on "Histopathology and Immunology of NHL". The audience did not seem familiar enough with the topic, so it was hard to reach them. In subsequent lectures, however, work done in Kiel was cited frequently by T. C. Brown (Toronto, Canada), D. M. V. Parrot (Glasgow, Scotland), and Lindberg (Lund, Sweden).

After the lectures I had a congenial lunch with Brown and Parrot. I found out that de Sousa had once worked with the latter. Then I spent some more time with Bettez, who had become a supporter of the Kiel classification since meeting me at a meeting of the International Academy of Pathology in Paris (see p. 40). Upon leaving I suggested that a central registry be established in Quebec where someone with knowledge of immunology would be available to everyone for consultation. There did not seem to be much interest in this idea, however.

de Champlain then drove with me to McGill University. She was a pathologist at the Jewish Hospital. Tremblay was waiting for us at the Institute of Pathology. He was one of about 30 pathologists in the department. I was asked to examine a case (sclerotic centroblastic-centrocytic lymphoma from the abdomen). Then I was given a tour. The Institute was proud of its teaching programme in small groups. De Champlain gave me slides from some interesting cases; the slides were of excellent histological quality.

2.16.6 JERUSALEM, 22–25 SEPTEMBER 1981

On 22 September I travelled on to Tel Aviv and from there to Jerusalem. Because of the meeting in Montreal I arrived late for the **Triennial World Congress of Societies of Pathology**.

On 23 September I met with Lukes to prepare our slide seminar. When we got to the lecture hall at the Institute of Pathology at Hadassah Medical School I was reminded of my visit there in 1976 (see p. 28). Polliack greeted me kindly. The audience was relatively small (40–50). My good friend LOPES-CARDOZO was there.

The next morning RENATE REIF and I moderated a session on lymphomas. As speakers we had invited S. POPPEMA (Hodgkin's disease), STEIN (immunohistology of B-cell lymphomas), T. SUCHI (malignant lymphomas in Japan), LUKES (immunoblastic lymphadenopathy), MEIJER (true histiocytic lymphoma), and RAMOT (Mediterranean intestinal lymphoma). The audience was so large that we had to move into a larger lecture hall. The session was said to be the best and the most popular one of the congress. During the break and afterwards I enjoyed conversations with RAMOT, DUHAMEL and his wife (from Paris), and MEÏR (from Strasbourg).

On 25 September LIFSCHITZ and his wife drove me to Tel Hashomer, where E. HERCZEG, J. J. BUBIS, and RAMOT were waiting for me. We spent a long time at the microscope discussing cases, all of which I was able to help clarify by explaining inflammatory lymph node lesions according to the principles of immunopathology. Then I gave a brief critical report on the Working Formulation and on angioimmunoblastic lymphadenopathy. RAMOT was very kind to me. I also enjoyed talking with HERCZEG, who told me what he thought of the political situation in Israel. He was discouraged because the Isrealis had not negotiated with the Arabs in 1967. Now it was too late because of oil. He also mentioned the conflict between Arabic and European Jews (similar to problems with African Americans in the USA). HERCZEG liked Germany very much and wanted to come as often as he could.

2.16.7 KIEL, 7–9 OCTOBER 1981

A **tutorial** was held in Kiel for Scandinavian pathologists to learn more about the diagnosis of NHL. SCHWARZE helped to organize it. The participants included 21 from Sweden, 10 from Denmark, five from Norway, and four from Finland. Material was submitted from Sweden (13 cases) and provided by the institute in Kiel (22 cases). The slides were examined under the microscope and jointly discussed with the aid of a video microscope. The atmosphere was very harmonious.

2.16.8 OXFORD, UK, 25–30 JANUARY 1982

On 25 January D. MASON and MORBELYN MOTA (from Venezuela) met me at the airport in London and drove me to Oxford for a **guest professorship**. J. MCGEE was my host at Linacre College of Oxford University. In the evening MOTA and I were invited for dinner at the home of MASON. MASON's wife was Danish and she tried speaking German with me. MOTA entertained us with Venezuelan songs and accompanied herself on a small guitar ("quadro"). The conversation centered around the problems of working wives.

The next day I visited MASON in his office. We were joined for discussion of cases by several others, including J. R. G. NASH (pathologist responsible for lymphomas), C. BARBATIS (pathologist), Z. ABDULAZIZ (from Iraq; prepared PAP stainings in MASON's laboratory), and K. C. GATTER. The latter worked with MASON and was impressed by my admitting when I did not know something. NASH presented the histological sections and MASON showed the corresponding immunohistochemical stainings. I was critical of the poor embedding technique and the lack of Giemsa staining. The discussion was tedious because of the poor slides, but I was still able to recognize some new features.

In the afternoon there was a macroscopic and microscopic demonstration of autopsy cases by remote video. This was impressive but took a long time. Then we went back to discussion at the microscope in MASON's office.

On 27 January MASON had organized a meeting on PAP staining results for my benefit so that I would have a larger audience. There were numerous presentations for about 80 listeners. The latter included BENNETT, MACLENNAN, WRIGHT, and P. G. ISAACSON. The talks were informal and interesting and some of the results were exciting. MCGEE left the meeting right after his presentation. JANOSSY mentioned in his talk that the handbook was a "bible". He presented a somewhat strange derivation scheme of the tumour cells of chronic lymphocytic leukaemia of B-cell type. I mentioned my doubts, but otherwise made few comments. All of the speakers used the terms of the Kiel classification. The atmosphere was very hospitable.

During the lunch break I enjoyed talking with MACLENNAN. He was an immunologist who had studied marginal zone cells with PAP staining. He was an enthusiastic supporter of the Kiel classification. STANSFELD introduced me to S. H. SWERDLOW, who had been working with COLLINS for two years and was especially interested in histiocytic and dendritic reticulum cells. I also had an opportunity to speak with BENNETT. He was doing a comprehensive study of 5,000 cases collected by the British lymphoma study group, starting with the cases of Hodgkin's disease.

Early in the evening I held a Litchfield Lecture. The topic was "Prelymphomas and Early Lymphomas" (myoepithelial sialadenitis, "lymphogranulomatosis X" [angioimmunoblastic lymphadenopathy]). I began by greeting ROBB-SMITH as the founder of the first lymph node registry in the world. Then I showed photographs of my most important co-workers and of the Institute of Pathology in Kiel in its three phases of development. I had some trouble with my English, but I was able to make a few jokes. WRIGHT told me later that he was impressed because I had shown photographs of my co-workers, which he thought was unusual. The lecture was followed by a 15-minute discussion and then by informal conversations that continued through dinner.

On 28 January I went to Blackwells, the famous bookshop in Oxford. I noticed that there were no German medical books for sale. In the afternoon I went on to the General Hospital in Southampton. WRIGHT greeted me there and showed me his department, where macroscopy was especially cultivated. I gave the same lecture I had given the day before, which WRIGHT thought went better this time, probably because I spoke freely. It was held in a small demonstration room (approx. 50 seats). WRIGHT was surprised at how full it was. In the evening I had dinner with five colleagues from WRIGHT's department; the conversation was not so pleasant when it turned to politics.

The next morning WRIGHT again took me to his department. The sign at the entrance said "D. Wright, Professor of Pathology" and not "Institute of Pathology". Evidently, departments of pathology were not desired. ISAACSON was there waiting for us. We discussed malignant "histiocytosis" of the intestine. ISAACSON told me about an interesting new finding in Mediterranean lymphoma, which he said was top secret. I was able to give him a few suggestions. With WRIGHT I discussed a case of nodular paragranuloma showing transformation into sarcoma after the course of several years.

The rest of the day WRIGHT took me sightseeing to Stonehenge and Salisbury. In the evening I returned to Oxford and met with MASON. As a haematologist he wished to cooperate with the Kiel research group, since he had no partners in pathology at Oxford. Then we had dinner with MCGEE and his wife, MOTA, and GATTER. The conversation was hearty and I enjoyed getting to know MCGEE better.

On the last day ROBB-SMITH and his wife took me to Woodstock to see Blenheim Castle, the birthplace of WINSTON CHURCHILL of whom ROBB-SMITH was very proud. Then they took me to their own house right next door for tea. The house had been built in the 12th century. ROBB-SMITH's large library was impressive.

In the evening I took a train to London to visit STANSFELD. We spoke about the future of the ELC. STANSFELD felt that the Club should continue and planned to write to VAN UNNIK. STANSFELD was very happy in retirement and had time to write a book on lymph node pathology.

The most remarkable observation that I made during my stay in the UK was the increasing acceptance of the Kiel classification. The British classification was subject to increasing criticism and the American classifications had hardly a chance in the UK.

2.16.9 USA, 25 FEBRUARY – 5 MARCH 1982

On my arrival in Rochester, MN on 25 February Banks was waiting for me at the airport. The next day I visited the **Mayo Clinic**. In the morning I was shown cases of T-cell lymphoma. The laboratory gave me some useful advice on techniques for frozen tissue to pass on to Stein.

In the afternoon I showed the colour transparencies I was planning to use in my lecture on T-cell lymphomas at the UCLA symposium (see below). The listeners were surprised at the diversity of T-cell lymphomas. I met K.K. Unni from Iceland, who had spent a year working with G. Dhom in Homburg/Saar, Germany. T. W. Morgan from Denver, CO was an enthusiast of the Kiel classification; he asked me to sign a copy of the handbook and send it to him.

The evening began with a cocktail party at the home of Banks. The other guests were Dahlin (bone pathologist) and his wife, Winckelmann (dermatologist who had attended the germinal centre conference in Kiel), R. V. Pierre (haematologist, specialized in preleukaemia), Li (histochemist), Morgan, several young assistants, and some technical assistants.

On 27 February Banks drove me to the airport. He suggested that I refrain from presenting the "classification" of T-cell lymphomas at the UCLA symposium because it would be too confusing.

From Rochester I travelled on to Squaw Valley, CA via Salt Lake City, UT and Reno, NV. Squaw Valley is a ski resort located in the mountains near Lake Tahoe. It is modelled after an Austrian or Bavarian village. The accommodations were quite primitive.

The **11th Annual UCLA Symposium** began with a buffet in the evening of 28 February. The topic of the symposium was "B and T Cell Tumors: Biological and Clinical Aspects" and it was organized by Ellen S. Vitetta [81]. That evening I enjoyed talking with Seligmann, who was now in politics, working for the French minister of culture. Then Schlossman came up to me. He wanted to make up for what had happened in Vienna the year before (see p. 68) and introduced me to the manager of the company that produced his new monoclonal antibodies so that I could obtain some new ones without delay. He also offered antibodies to J. A. Habeshaw, with whom I had a nice conversation.

On 1 March I got up early to prepare my colour transparencies for the lecture since I suspected that there would be technical problems similar to ones

I had had in the USA before (known as the "carousel phenomenon"[3]). The symposium took place in the primitive "theatre". The co-authors of my presentation were STEIN, FELLER, and J. GERDES [82]. In the introduction I made some friendly remarks to SCHLOSSMAN. I presented the results of analyses of T-cell lymphomas, including innumerable tracings of nuclei in photographs. In most cases the nuclei proved to be distinctly pleomorphic (including a "jellyfish-like" type). In addition I presented numerous immunohistochemical findings. I also described Lennert's lymphoma and its differential diagnosis. For special effect I mentioned a lymphoma that later turned out to be Ki-1+ and went into remission in response to chemotherapy; a remarkable feature of the latter development was that the tumour cells became smaller. The audience did not seem to take much notice of this and other remarks, but there was much applause.

ROSENBERG reported on the results of the NCI study and ended his lecture by repeating his opinion that all six lymphoma classifications are of equal value. I spent the rest of the afternoon and evening with HABESHAW.

The lectures in the morning of the second day of the symposium were of high quality. P. H. KRAMMER gave an excellent presentation. He was planning to leave Heidelberg, Germany and work in the USA.

In the afternoon there was a workshop on lymphoma classifications moderated by JAFFE and WARNKE. Unfortunately, the workshop went poorly. JAFFE presented her hypothesis that follicular lymphoma is benign, since there are no other benign lymphomas. I disagreed and said that her reasoning was wrong. I pointed out benign lymphoma of the rectum as an example.

After the workshop I enjoyed conversations with BLOOMFIELD. I also had a long and friendly talk with GAJL-PECZALSKA. She was doing immunohistochemical analyses of malignant lymphomas together with BLOOMFIELD and FRIZZERA [83]. They had been using 13 antibodies on single cell suspensions and frozen sections. The results obtained in 100 cases largely corresponded to our findings, even though the nomenclature was different (the group in Minneapolis used the Working Formulation).

In the evening I had another conversation with HABESHAW. Like JAFFE he thought that follicular lymphoma was benign and often polyclonal. I dis-

3 Colour transparencies that are not framed in cardboard often get jammed or will not fit in most slide projectors used in the USA (known as "carousels"). Fortunately, this time I had brought my own projector. This made it possible for me to show my own transparencies and also to help out a few other speakers from Europe who otherwise would have had the same problem.

agreed and mentioned that GAJL-PECZALSKA had also found only monoclonal lymphomas of this type. We got into a heated argument. Nevertheless, HABESHAW was not offended and we parted cordially.

On 3 March the owner of the ski lodge, W. PARSON, and his wife invited me to lunch. They spoke German since he had been born in Transylvania and she in Austria. They were very kind to me.

In the afternoon there was a well-organized and stimulating session on B-cell and T-cell lymphoma markers moderated by BLOOMFIELD. Afterwards G.E. MARTI joined me for supper and we had a nice conversation. MARTI was an immunogeneticist who used to work in Chicago and was now at the NIH in Bethesda, MD. I gave him a copy of our recent book [60] since he had shown so much interest in morphology and had admired the high quality of the histological and histochemical slides I had presented.

On 4 March the lectures were not of great interest to me (e.g. animal pathology). There was one presentation that stood out, however, namely that given by M. FELDMAN. He was a very dynamic speaker.

In the afternoon the participants went to the top of one of the mountains by gondola. Here I had an opportunity for many conversations. FELDMAN came up to me and asked about the continuous Hodgkin cell lines of KAPLAN. FELDMAN believed in them, whereas I was sceptical. He mentioned interest in visiting Kiel. I also spoke briefly with WALDMANN. He praised my lecture and said it was good to meet me after hearing so much about me. I told him that his lecture was the highlight of the symposium.

On the last day there were several more cordial encounters. WARNKE, for example, looked forward to visiting me in Kiel. I also had a few final words with SELIGMANN.

In retrospect, I wondered why there were not more than 10 "old warriors" from the lymphoma battlefield. Had they not been invited? Where was my generation? There were about 300 young people there, however, who were very lively.

2.16.10 COPENHAGEN, DENMARK, 28–30 JUNE 1982

The **Nordic Congress of Pathological Anatomy and Cytology** was the first pathology congress for all four Scandinavian countries. There were about 250 participants. The congress was held in English to accommodate the Finns. My slide seminar on reactive lymph node lesions was scheduled at the end of the congress in order to keep people from leaving early. The congress secretary, B. HAINAU, gave ingenious and polished opening remarks. He emphasized the necessity to learn from German pathology and mentioned R. VIRCHOW, ASCHOFF, D.P. HANSEMANN, and SANDRITTER. In the seminar

I demonstrated plasmacytoid T cells for the first time and a case of Kikuchi's lymphadenitis caused by Yersinia enterocolitica. The seminar went well, even though the atmosphere was somewhat strained. The audience was very attentive. The participants included a few old friends, but most of them were "newcomers".

At breakfast I enjoyed a conversation with A. TALERMAN. After the seminar HAINAU invited me to his home, where I met his wife who came from Berlin. I also enjoyed speaking with the president of the congress, S. OLSEN, and his wife. He was professor of pathology in Aarhus, specializing in renal pathology, and a friend of A. BOHLE. OLSEN remembered visiting me in 1958 in Frankfurt a. M., where I gave him material from a case of Masshoff's lymphadenitis, which made this disease known in Denmark.

2.16.11 FREIBURG, GERMANY, 6 JULY 1982

The Faculty of Medicine at the University of Freiburg awarded me the **Aschoff Medal**. I was asked to give a lecture at the ceremony.

The topic of my lecture in the evening of 6 July was prelymphomas and early lymphomas, which I had spoken about in a presentation at the Congress of the German Society of Pathology in 1979. The lecture hall in Freiburg was overfilled and very hot. About 70% of the audience were students and many members of the faculty were there. BÜCHNER and SANDRITTER's wife were sitting in the first row. In my introductory remarks I reminisced about my faithful friend SANDRITTER, who had died in 1980. There was a lump in my throat and the audience was absolutely silent. Then I went on with the lecture as usual, which was received with hearty applause. The Dean presented me with the silver Aschoff Medal, which had been instituted by the Faculty of Medicine at the suggestion of SANDRITTER. The inscription read *"Leben heißt arbeiten"* (translation: to live means to work), which was obviously a quotation from ASCHOFF.

The next day was SANDRITTER's birthday. His wife, my wife and I visited his grave.

2.16.12 KIEL, 2–6 AUGUST 1982

NANCY L. HARRIS (Boston) spent a week working with me. She was surprised by the hospitality and by the number of guests at the Lymph Node Registry. WARNKE also came to Kiel for a few days and gave a lecture. At the time PIRIS (from Spain) was working at the Institute of Pathology in Kiel.

2.16.13 SEATTLE, WA, USA, 6–7 SEPTEMBER 1982

All the sessions at **The Second Seminar on Differences in Lymphocytic Diseases in the US and Japan** were moderated by BERARD. Unfortunately, he did not have time for a conversation with me. I did not want to surprise him and would have liked to tell him that I was not going to agree to the Working Formulation at the UICC Cancer Congress a few days later (see pp. 57ff.).

The introductory lecture was held by B. MILLER of the NIH. He presented the results of an epidemiologic comparison of lymphomas and other diseases (including rheumatoid diseases) in Japan and the USA. The other presentations were of varying quality. Surprisingly, MOHRI presented his own lymphoma classification, which was a combination of the Kiel classification and the WHO classification (!).

The most important topic was T-cell lymphoma, especially ATLL. Presentations were given by HANAOKA, KIKUCHI, SUCHI, and K. TAKATSUKI. The latter was an internist who used excellent immunological techniques and evidently discovered ATLL [84]. CATOVSKY reported on ATLL in Blacks from the West Indies. KADIN reported on nonendemic ATLL in six Caucasian patients. J.W. SAID presented ultrastructural findings; he had a large collection of cases and worked with GERALDINE S. PINKUS. M. SHIMOYAMA [29] gave a talk on "T-cell lymphoma with suppressor/cytotoxic T-cell phenotype", which corresponded to what I defined at the time as lymphogranulomatosis X [26,27]. He thought it was a malignant T-cell tumour, however, whereas I said it was a nonneoplastic lesion. ALEXANDRA LEVINE spoke about T-immunoblastic lymphoma.

The talk I gave on T-cell lymphomas was the last one on the first evening of the seminar. It was the first time that I presented plasmacytoid T-cell lymphoma. I also described T-zone lymphoma, pleomorphic T-cell lymphoma, and lymphoepithelioid lymphoma (Lennert's lymphoma). There was much confusion over the latter. In the early 1970s it had become clear that it was not "simply Hodgkin's disease"; many cases proved to be T-cell lymphomas.

Viral induced lymphoproliferative diseases in immunodeficient patients was the topic of a presentation by D. PURTILO. STEIN presented the immunohistology of Hodgkin's disease. WAKASA and DORFMAN described necrotizing lymphadenitis (also known as Kikuchi's lymphadenitis). KOJIMA spoke about multicentric lymphadenopathy histologically simulating Castleman's disease.

During the discussions BERARD kept asking me to make comments. I lost my patience and said that I did not want to appear to be the "Pope". Finally, he demanded that I express my opinion on the Working Formulation. I explained that I rejected the Working Formulation because it did not define biological entities. BERARD contradicted me. I had already informed O'CONOR and DORFMAN of my criticism.

In the evening I had dinner with MOHRI, KIKUCHI, and STEIN. I asked MOHRI about his classification. Was it pure opportunism, weakness, or insecurity? STEIN said that he would have to bear the ridicule and he and KIKUCHI laughed at him. I was horrified that MOHRI had spent five years in Kiel and studied thousands of cases classified by the Kiel classification and had now thrown everything overboard.

The next day I went on a boat trip with STEIN to Victoria, Canada, where we visited the Butchart Gardens. On the boat STEIN talked about his departure for Oxford, UK on 1 November 1982. He would be turning his laboratory over to FELLER. Following his stay in the UK STEIN would be moving to Berlin.

NATHWANI and his wife were also on the boat. We had some scientific arguments. NATHWANI said that he respected the work done in Kiel and the handbook in particular, but on some topics he was of a different opinion. He mentioned a positive example: the pseudofollicular proliferation centres in chronic lymphocytic leukaemia permit a diagnosis within seconds. I told him that I was very sad because of the animosities towards me that had arisen in the USA. I invited him to come to Kiel and see for himself what we were doing in our laboratories. He planned to apply for a grant from the German Academic Exchange Service (DAAD). NATHWANI was a fiery man who worked under RAPPAPORT at the City of Hope Cancer Center in Duarte, CA, USA. He told me that the immunological techniques used at the Cancer Center were primitive. The Center received only about 300 new cases per year, but did see many cases for consultation (approx. 2,000 per year). About 100 autopsies were performed at the Center and there were approx. 3,000–5,000 biopsies in all per year.

2.16.14 BIRMINGHAM, UK, 20 SEPTEMBER 1982

The **Birmingham International Symposium on Head and Neck Cancer** was held in a chemistry lecture hall. Humorous introductory remarks were given by P. BEVAN, a surgeon. The lecture hall was only about half full and most of the approx. 100 listeners were clinicians who did not appear to understand us pathologists. I was introduced by R. BROWN, an oral pathologist from Birmingham. He asked an odd question about myoepithelial complexes in Sjögren's syndrome. In my lecture I presented the pathology of cervical lymph nodes, Waldeyer's ring (including findings of RILKE), and the salivary glands [85]. D. F. N. HARRISON (director of the Department of Oral Surgery) criticized me sharply and said that "low grade" and "high grade" depend on stage of the disease and treatment and not on morphology. E. WILLIAMS gave a very good lecture on tumours of the thyroid gland. He invited me to visit him in Cardiff, Wales.

After the symposium I had a good conversation with G. DE THÉ on the way to the airport. He mentioned that about 3,000 of the 7,000 participants at the meeting in Seattle two weeks previously (see pp. 56ff.) were from Japan.

STANSFELD and I had arranged to meet at the airport. I was glad to see him and to exchange views after the meeting in Seattle. STANSFELD was firmly opposed to the Working Formulation. He reported on bad experiences with the British National Health System and said that more and more people were choosing private insurance. He though that the German health system was probably better.

The next day I noticed that the Working Formulation was occupying my mind more than the upcoming trip to South America.

2.16.15 BRAZIL, 22–26 SEPTEMBER 1982

In São Paulo I was met at the airport by SCHWARZE and two of MACHADO's assistants, G. S. HIDALGO and A. C. ALVES. I was allowed through customs quickly because I was a "professor". At the hotel I met two Brazilians, J. VERCELLI and P. PAES, as they were also inquiring about the arrival of DIEBOLD. PAES had spent a year working with DIEBOLD in Paris. PAES and I had lunch together and I told him about the Working Formulation and the meeting in Seattle. The result of our conversation was that PAES changed his opinion of the Rappaport and Kiel classifications. Beforehand he had defended the former against the latter. Afterwards he became a supporter of the Kiel classification. In the evening I had dinner with MACHADO and his wife, SCHWARZE, and DIEBOLD.

The **Latin American Club for Haematopathology** and the **National** (Brazilian) **Commission for Malignant Lymphomas** held a symposium in São Paulo, 23–25 September. The participants included S. BESUSCHIO, P. A. ROLON (who later came to Kiel for three months), MACHADO, ROESCH (who later came to Kiel for 12 months), LORAND (who had already been in Kiel for six months in 1977/78), E. CHAVES, and DE CASTRO (who came to Kiel several times). The symposium took place at the *Instituto Butantan*, where research on snake poisons was done. There was also a department of pathology, of which MACHADO was still director. He was also director of the Institute of Pathology at the cancer hospital. The *Instituto Butantan* had set up a room with 20 microscopes for the participants. On the wall there were photographs of all the previous meetings of lymphoma experts, including our first tutorial in 1976 (see p. 31).

The symposium was held in a small lecture hall with seats for a maximum of 100 listeners. It was so full that some people had to stand. My old friend JAMRA was there. He wanted to help me to get LORAND's Portuguese translation of the lymphoma book published (unfortunately with no success). At the symposium I was asked to report on the pathology of T-cell lymphomas. After my presentation DIEBOLD gave a comprehensive and systematic review of splenic lymphomas and other types of splenomegaly. In the afternoon there was a seminar on the spleen. I spent the evening with the South American lymphoma club and Brazilian lymphoma experts. They were all supporters of the Kiel classification.

The next morning I held a slide seminar on lymphoma-like lymph node lesions. The participants were disappointed that there was only one who could recognize the case of leishmaniasis that I presented. The atmosphere was friendly, but it was not easy to discuss all 18 slides in just two hours.

There was a round table discussion in the afternoon, moderated by MACHADO. The speakers were DIEBOLD, BESUSCHIO, and myself. BESUSCHIO declared his support of the Kiel classification and had just three small difficulties with it that I was able to clarify easily. For example, he asked why immature plasmacytoma was not included in the Kiel classification. His comments on the Working Formulation were: "The result is very poor in relation to the magnitude of the task" and "Also this work was wrong for creating ideas". DIEBOLD's support was very eloquent and spontaneous. I reported on the current status of the Kiel classification, including recent clinical and immunological findings, and on the disastrous meeting in Seattle (see pp. 57ff.). This evoked hearty applause. In the evening MACHADO held a reception at his new appartment.

In the morning of 25 September SCHWARZE held a seminar on lymphoma cytology as shown by smears. Then I went on a tour of the city with DIEBOLD. Later I flew on to Rio de Janeiro together with DIEBOLD and DE CASTRO. During dinner with DIEBOLD he told me about the situation of pathologists in Paris. He was having problems with SELIGMANN, who was now working for the government, but these were due to his being dean of the medical faculty. DIEBOLD and L. ORCEL were the only tenured professors of pathology in Paris. DIEBOLD was not only dean, but also president of all the medical deans in Paris. He had much respect for NÉZELOF and tried to help him whenever he could.

The next day DE CASTRO met me and DIEBOLD and drove us through the city to a boat that took us out to the small island where DE CASTRO lived (to be safe from burglars). Many family friends and guests were there. DE CASTRO kept up with current research and was a full supporter of the Kiel classification. After a sumptuous meal he drove us to the airport to catch our aeroplanes back to Europe.

In retrospect I noted the following in my diary. The Brazilian population makes up about half the total population of South America. Brazil is the most modern nation there. There are about 500 pathologists in Brazil, while all other countries together have only about 200. I noticed that enormous progress had been made in the diagnosis of lymph node diseases. For example, all of the participants in the seminar had recognized infectious mononucleosis. In Germany perhaps about half of the participants would have diagnosed malignant lymphoma.

Besuschio, who came from Argentina, was also an excellent pathologist and an enthusiastic supporter of the Kiel classification. He worked with A. Pavlovsky in Buenos Aires. He was planning to turn the international haematopathology congress (in 1984) into a success for the Kiel classification. In his lecture at the symposium he cited the philosophers R. Descartes and J. Ortega y Gasset.

Machado did much for the Kiel classification in South America. The first spark was struck by Jamra, however, with whom I had become friends in London (see p. 26) and who had prompted Machado to attend the tutorial in Damp in 1975 (see p. 28). Machado was a firm supporter of the Kiel classification and founded the South American lymphoma club, of which Diebold was also a member (Fig. 14). How efficient was the club? The members met about once a year and evidently exchanged slides. The clinicians caused problems for the supporters of the Kiel classification because (a) there

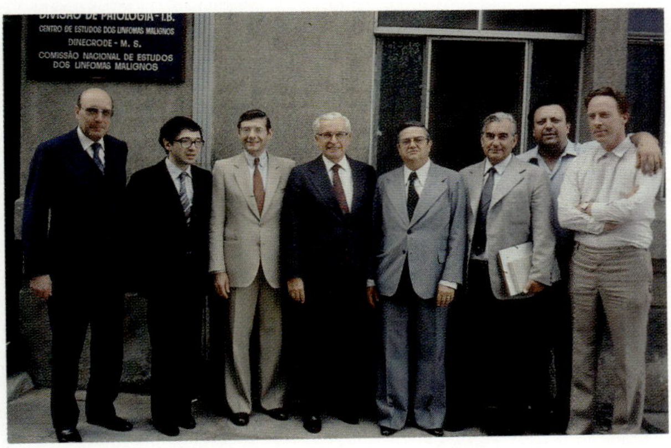

Fig. 14 Members of the South American Lymphoma Club in São Paulo, Brazil, 1982. *Left to right:* S. Besuschio, G. Varcelli, J. Diebold, the author, J.C. Machado (initiator of cooperation with South America), P.A. Rolon, H. Navarette, J. Rohmann

were no treatment guidelines and (b) the hospitals were dependent on grants from the USA and therefore required to use the Working Formulation. I thought we should send treatment protocolls to the club.

Rolon from Paraguay made a particularly good impression on me. He was an experienced pathologist who was very knowledgeable in many fields, including politics.

2.16.16 ROME, ITALY, 3–6 OCTOBER 1982

At the suggestion of Rilke, I was invited to hold a course on lymphoma pathology at the Catholic University in Rome, which belongs to the Vatican. I was officially invited by P. Donnorso, a cytopathologist. He was a lively man, a very good organizer, and a gracious host.

The course went well, but I had no personal contact with the participants because they did not understand English and the translation was not simultaneous. Rilke helped where he could. My presentation lasted all morning and took place in a grandiose lecture hall. In the afternoon the participants could use microscopes in five rooms; this was supervised by Rilke. At the end of the course all of the participants were satisfied. Many of them expressed interest in coming to Kiel themselves or sending assistants. Mirella Marino was one of them and she later came to Kiel twice for several months.

2.16.17 1983

At a number of congresses in 1983 a comprehensive presentation of the classification of lymphomas was at the focus of attention, especially in German-speaking countries. The possibility that T-cell lymphomas are induced by viruses was discussed at several meetings. This was also the year that I met Anna Tu (see p. 87) and learned about the Chinese views on lymphoma classification.

2.16.17.1 WIESBADEN, GERMANY, 14 APRIL 1983

At the **89th Meeting of the German Society of Internal Medicine** one of the main topics was malignant lymphomas. The session on Hodgkin's disease and NHL was moderated by H.J. Dengler and myself. The topic of my lecture was the pathology of NHL. Other lectures were given by R. Fischer, Diehl, Löffler, Brittinger, Theml, and Rühl.

2.16.17.2 LUCERNE, SWITZERLAND, 24–28 MAY 1983

Since, as president, I was responsible for organizing the **67th Meeting of the German Society of Pathology** [86] I took the liberty of choosing just one main topic, namely haematopathology. Virtually all fields of morphological haematopathology were discussed for five whole days. At the end of the meeting half of one day was devoted to NHL, with lectures by STEIN, BRITTINGER, and others. The discussion of T-cell lymphomas received a new impulse from the discovery of HTLV-positive lymphomas in Japan. This led us to organize a special workshop on the topic (see below).

2.16.17.3 KIEL, 5–11 SEPTEMBER 1983

A **workshop** was held to discuss **European HTLV-negative and Japanese HTLV-positive T-cell lymphomas**. The Japanese participants were E. SATO, SUCHI, and KIKUCHI. The European participants were STANSFELD, FELLER, GÖDDE-SALZ, M. L. HANSMANN, MÜLLER-HERMELINK, and myself (Fig. 15). A total of 18 HTLV-positive and 31 HTLV-negative cases were examined.

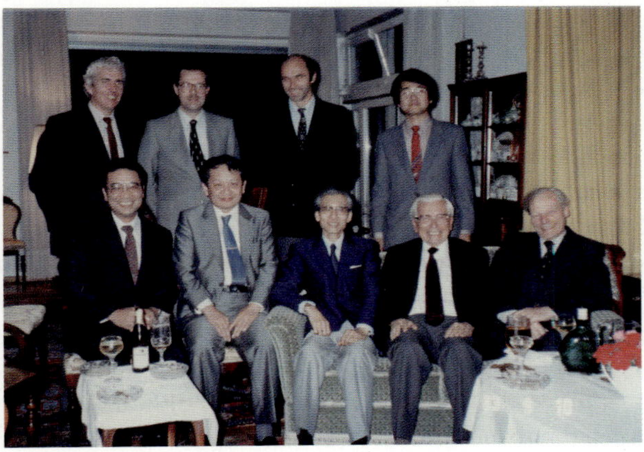

Fig. 15 Participants in the Japanese-German workshop on virus-induced T-cell lymphomas in Japan in comparison with virus-negative European T-cell lymphomas, Kiel, Germany, 1983. *First row, left to right:* E. SATO, M. KIKUCHI, T. SUCHI, the author, A. G. STANSFELD. *Second row:* H. K. MÜLLER-HERMELINK, M.-L. HANSMANN, A. C. FELLER, K. HASUI

They were classified as pleomorphic (peripheral) T-cell lymphomas with tumour cells of various sizes [87]. In a blind trial KIKUCHI and SATO were able to morphologically identify 80% of HTLV-positive cases.

2.16.17.4 COLD SPRING HARBOR, NY, USA, 14–15 SEPTEMBER 1983

Immediately after the workshop in Kiel a symposium entitled **"Human T- Cell Leukemia Viruses"** was organized by M. ESSEX and GALLO in the USA. The accommodations were primitive. My roommates were GALLO and CATOVSKY. In the morning before the meeting I was able to have a conversation with GALLO. He did not accept my suggestion to report on the results of the German-Japanese workshop in Kiel. He said that I could mention them in my introductory remarks as chairman of the evening session.

The symposium was run informally. Most of the participants were between 25 and 40 years old. The only "oldsters" were KAPLAN, GROSS, and myself. GROSS described the mouse leukaemias that had been induced by a virus. He had received the Paul Ehrlich prize and wore a medal of the French Legion of Honour. I told him that I had been citing his work for 30 years when I was teaching.

There were many participants from Japan. M. YOSHIDA seemed to be the best one. It was obvious that there was animosity between the Japanese and the Americans. HTLV was new on the market. In retrospect I could understand why GALLO did not want to hear about the German-Japanese study. The Japanese presentations were excellent. There were also 10 talks given by employees of the NIH. There were no speakers from Germany. I was the only invited guest from Germany. Many of the Americans were German, however, and they greeted me kindly. These included P. VOGT (from Los Angeles) and P.H. DUESBERG (a virologist from Berkeley, CA). M.A. LUTZNER had returned to the NIH from Paris. There was not one morphological presentation, as I criticized in my introduction to the evening session. I thought that morphology was underestimated. GALLO, however, felt that morphology was not opportune in Cold Spring Harbor. Although my introductory remarks were applauded, they were understood by only a few (e.g. N.L. WARNER). GALLO did not show much interest, even though he was very friendly in private. Another Japanese participant was Y. ITO (from Kyoto). GREAVES approached me for the first time. CATOVSKY was more friendly than the last time we met. He told me that he had held six lectures at the African-European congress of the International Society of Haematology. He was impressed by the presentation given there by H.J. RADZUN of the Institute of Pathology in Kiel.

2.16.17.5 HAMBURG, GERMANY, 19–24 SEPTEMBER 1983

At the **9th Congress of the European Society of Pathology** I held the Symeonides lecture, which was entitled "New Aspects in the Research of Lymphomas". I did not give an introduction to the Kiel classification, but instead presented "new aspects". I reported on the results of the German-Japanese study and of immunological analyses by the research group in Kiel in cases of T-cell lymphoma, especially ATLL. I also mentioned recent data showing the clinical relevance of the Kiel classification.

2.16.17.6 LONDON, 29–30 SEPTEMBER 1983

Stansfeld organized a **meeting of the ELC**. At this meeting Anna Tu was accepted as an honorary member of the club. We looked at a large number of histological slides. I demonstrated the first case of malignant lymphoma of monocytoid B cells that we had been able to identify as such.

After the meeting Tu accompanied me to Kiel. She had spent a year working with Bennett in the UK. At the time she was employed at the Institute of Pathology in Shanghai. She had a difficult time walking and had to use a cane, supposedly because of arthrosis. Later it was discovered that she had carcinoma of the colon with bone metastases.

2.16.17.7 KIEL, 1–7 OCTOBER 1983

At Tu's request she stayed in the guest room at the Institute of Pathology because she wanted to spend as much time as possible at the microscope and discussing cases with me. Together we examined the Japanese series. Tu noticed a new type of lymphoma composed of medium-sized basophilic cells. We drafted a scheme of T-cell lymphomas that Tu would take to Suchi.

While she was in Kiel Tu did hardly anything besides work. We spent many hours together at the microscope. She had excellent eyes and a good mind. She was very grateful for everything and we became good friends.

2.16.17.8 BOLOGNA, ITALY, 17–18 OCTOBER 1983

S. Pileri organized a meeting on **"Current Topics in Lymphopathology"**. P. P. Piccaluga and I functioned merely as "presidents". Most of the presentations were given by Italians. There were a few speakers from Kiel, including

M. L. GEERTS and U. SCHMID. One of the topics was T-cell lymphoma. I was asked to comment on the Working Formulation. The atmosphere was very friendly and most of the pariticipants were supporters of the Kiel classification.

2.16.17.9 MOROCCO, 23–26 OCTOBER 1983

Under the auspices of the Goethe Institute MÜLLER-HERMELINK and I were invited to give a **slide demonstration on malignant lymphomas** at the institute of G. GUERBAOUI in **Casablanca**. He was a Berber who had spent 16 years in Strasbourg. He and his Alsation wife and WÄBER of the Goethe Institute met us at the airport. The lectures and demonstrations given by MÜLLER-HERMELINK (in French) and myself (in English) were not very effective because the listeners did not have enough background knowledge.

We also visited the institute in **Rabat**, which was much larger and very well equipped. Unfortunately, the 10 assistants had very little knowledge of how to use the equipment. For example, an electron microscope that had been donated from Europe had never been unpacked. There was only one laboratory assistant and one secretary.

On the last evening of our stay GUERBAOUI hosted a festive dinner at his apartment, with roast mutton and couscous. The hospitality of the Moroccans was overwhelming.

2.16.18 1984

The most significant event in 1984 was my first trip to China, where I gave several seminars and lectures that were translated by TU. There was great interest in the Kiel classification in China. Unfortunately, the cooperation between Kiel and China did not develop to the planned degree because of the tragic death of TU in 1986.

The same year I also visited Japan, South America, and the USA. The pathology of T-cell lymphomas was the focus of most presentations. The year began with a lecture in France and ended with a stimulating symposium in Siena, Italy, followed by a gratifying stay in Birmingham, UK.

2.16.18.1 FRANCE, 26–28 APRIL 1984

On 26 April I held a lecture on malignant lymphomas in **Lyon**. I enjoyed meeting FRANÇOISE BERGER.

J. J. SOTTO organized a seminar on NHL in **Grenoble**, 27–28 April. The evening before the seminar I had dinner with LUKES, who did not seem well. The next morning LUKES, DIEBOLD, and I each held a lecture on the classification of NHL. DIEBOLD commented in detail on the Working Formulation, in much the critical way I would have done. That evening I joined BRITTINGER and his wife, H. RIEHM, and WRIGHT. WRIGHT was very active in China supporting the Kiel classification. His opinion of the current political situation in China was positive. RIEHM expressed his regret that he had become aware of the immunological concept of the Kiel classification so late. I had to leave the next morning, but the seminar continued with presentations by WRIGHT, AUDOUIN, PANGALIS, TUBIANA, BRITTINGER, MATHÉ, and others.

2.16.18.2 CHINA, 29 APRIL – 12 MAY 1984

In **Beijing** my wife and I were met by TU and her colleague HU, who were our gracious hosts and guides during our stay. The hotel where we stayed first used to be the residence of a higher pre-communist official. The day after our arrival we had an opportunity to visit the Chinese Wall.

On 3 May I gave a lecture at the Institute of Cancer Research in Beijing. The director was GNA, 58 years old, who had spent four postgraduate years in Leningrad. In 1983 he had spent a few months in the USA. He had also been in East Germany for 1½ months. He knew a lot about oncogenes and laser therapy. His assistant CHANG was very helpful in preparing everything for my lecture, which was held in a primitive lecture hall with a small blackboard and a small slide screen. There were about 100 listeners, approx. 80% of them were pathologists. Some of them were wearing uniform caps. TU translated my lecture.

In my lecture I began by showing photographs of the Institute of Pathology in Kiel and of my co-workers, who sent friendly greetings to their Chinese colleagues and who remembered meeting TU the previous year. We hoped that the contact between Kiel and Beijing could be intensified. Then I showed a table comparing the six classifications of NHL in current use. They were the ones compared in the NCI study, on the basis of survival data. Those data were not adequate for evaluating a classification. One of the most important criteria is the compatibility of a classification with the modern immune system (B and T cells). This was realized only in the Lukes-Collins and Kiel classifications. LUKES had presented his classification in China the previous year. Now it was my turn. The Kiel classification was not the accomplishment of a single person, but rather a collaborative effort from the very beginning. I showed photographs of the members of the ELC, who developed the basic concept of the Kiel classification in Kiel almost exactly 10 years previously (see pp. 18ff.). Soon a retrospective study and then a large prospective clinical study were initiated by STACHER and then carried on under the leadership of BRITTINGER. It soon became evident that the Kiel classification was not an artefact, but that it defined entities with correspondingly distinct clinical features [38]. By 1984 the Kiel classification had become widely accepted in Europe. The European Lymphoma Study Group (a group composed of about 80–100 European pathologists; see p. 112) met once every two years at a workshop for training in the diagnosis of lymphomas according to the Kiel classification. I mentioned that the ELC had accepted TU as an honorary member at its last meeting in London (see p. 87) in order to document the bond between European and Chinese medicine, which we hoped would become even stronger in the future.

The lecture lasted for 2½ hours with a break of only five minutes, but I was provided with a pot of green tea to refresh myself. The audience was partially interested and partially bored. A few people even fell asleep. One particularly interested listener asked me about the nature of angioimmunoblastic lymphadenopathly with dysproteinaemia (AILD); he seemed to know what he was talking about. The lecture went well, and at the end I invited the audience to cooperate with other countries. China had tremendous opportunities with its huge amount of material for research.

After the lecture GNA invited TU, HU, and my wife and myself to a dinner of Peking duck. When we got back to the hotel we found out that we had to move to another, more modern hotel.

Early the next morning HU picked us up and took us to Tiän tan Hospital, where ZHU CHANG REN was head of the department of pathology. We arrived late and found ZHU waiting in the park. He was a fine gray-haired man who had translated parts of my first handbook while he was exiled during the Cultural Revolution. He gave me his last copy of the book, which looked like a thick pamphlet. Years later he apologized for translating the book without asking me and drew a calligraphic scroll for me as compensation. Eventually he moved to the USA to be with his two sons. When we met in Beijing he expressed interest in visiting Kiel. He showed us what he thought was the most beautiful temple in China (the "Heavenly Temple") and the 300 year old cedars in the park.

That afternoon we left for **Xi'an**. At the airport we were met by a large group of people: LIU YAN-FANG, SHUI SU HUA, YUNG DIN-TONG, YANG SHAO-VAN, and three others. LIU was a professor of pathology at the IV. Military College. He was about 60 years old and spoke English well; he had been a translator for Americans in about 1940. TU thought it was very important that I accept his invitation. He organized our visit in Xi'an and was a friendly host. SHUI was the head pathologist at the Central Hospital. She had been a student of TU's. YUNG was a professor of medicine at the I. College and vice-president of the regional pathology society. YANG was a nice young co-worker of LIU's.

At the hotel we were given a large appartment with two rooms and a bath. After a snack LIU took us on a tour of the city. He showed us an old mosque and a drum tower. From the tower we could see many poor houses that were being torn down or renovated. The two-story houses were so different from Beijing.

After dinner LIU's assistant YANG came to discuss the rest of our visit. We were later joined by my translator, SHE LE-CHENG, and a pathology professor from I. Medical College to prepare for my lectures the next day.

The next morning LIU took us to visit a museum (history of China) that had a large collection of stelae. Lunch was a large meal with eight bowls of food (and chopsticks). Afterwards it turned out that I had to pay for everything: the hotel, meals, rental car, and guides. The total cost was exorbitant.

In the afternoon LIU took us to the lecture hall, which was overfilled. There were about 100 pathologists, most of whom were young and dressed in uniforms with caps on their heads. There were also a few grey-haired colleagues. I had been asked to give two lectures, one on the Kiel classification and one on immunohistochemistry of NHL. After the first lecture (1½ hours) there was a 10-minute break. Then everyone came back for the second lecture (another 1½ hours). In contrast to Beijing there were no problems with the slide projection. LIU found my presentations convincing and intended to support the Kiel classification. He seemed to be very knowledgeable and interested in immunology.

After the lectures we visited a civilian institute of pathology, which was simple and clean. A cryostat and monoclonal antibodies were in use. We were shown only two laboratories and not allowed into the autopsy room. Anatomical specimens were displayed in the halls. We were told that about 80 autopsies were performed and 7,000 biopsies were examined each year. This was comparable to the volume at the military institute.

In the evening the faculty held a dinner for us, at which there were some short speeches and we were given a terracotta horse. Afterwards I went for a walk by myself and got lost when the front door of a store was locked and I was forced to leave by the back door. No one on the streets understood me. Finally, a young girl understood "hotel" and showed me the way back. There was still lots of merchant activity on the streets. I got a glimpse of some sleeping quarters: 10 beds one behind the other. The people slept fully dressed with no sheets or blankets.

On 6 May YANG CHANG HUA (a student) and his wife picked us up to go to see the terracotta soldiers at the tomb of the first emperor of China, QIN SHI HUANG (259–210 B.C.). We stopped at the Huaqing Hot Springs near Mt. Lishan, where the escape of CHIANG KAI-SHEK was described in full detail. He had hidden there. There were bullet holes in the bedroom. YANG's wife was very friendly but not willing to discuss politics.

After another sumptuous lunch we were taken shopping, but we did not buy anything. Later at the airport the same large group of people who had met us were there to say farewell. They were very helpful getting us and our luggage onto the aeroplane.

That evening we arrived in **Shanghai**, where TU and XU LIANG ZHONG were waiting for us. XU was a cytogeneticist who had worked in Southampton, UK and at the NCI. A limousine took us to a guest house where we had a large room with bath. Flowers had been put on the table for my wife because it was Mother's Day.

The next morning ZHANG HUA ZHONG met us and took us to the temple of the jade Buddha. ZHANG was half Chinese, half Indonesian. After the Revolution he left Indonesia and chose to come to China. He worked with XU. Previously he had spent one year working with the cytologist SU and two years with JAFFE at the NCI in Washington, DC. He had analyzed lymphomas with the avidin method.

In the evening we were invited to a banquet with about 12 dignitaries. The most honoured guest was GU, an emeritus professor of pathology. He was highly regarded by everyone and treated like royalty by younger colleagues. He suffered from the effects of a stroke. He was very kind and genuinely pleased to meet us. The other guests were leading pathologists. One of them was LU YI YU, the director of the Cancer Institute. He had visited the German Cancer Research Centre in Heidelberg and had attended the gastroenterology congress in Mainz. He seemed to be very skilled in his field and resolute, but at the same time friendly and modest. XU and TU were also there, but neither of them said anything. LU proposed the first toast and I responded, whereby he stood and I had to sit down. The atmosphere was very friendly and the meal was excellent. Some of the guests were dressed in the European style.

In the morning of 8 May ZHANG took us on a tour of the city. In the afternoon I gave a 2½-hour lecture on NHL, including immunohistochemistry, which was again translated by TU. I was introduced by HO. GU insisted on attending even though he was not well. After the first half of the lecture he left, however, escorted by some of his students.

TU graciously invited us to her home in the evening. Everything was very simple. TU had five children, born while she was in the USA. At the time of our visit three of them had returned to the USA, another would follow soon. TU's husband was a surgeon and a member of the General Assembly. He had trained in the USA. Her father had also been in the USA, where he received a PhD, and he spoke four languages. During the Cultural Revolution he was put into prison and went insane. Every day he was told to confess that he was a conspirator until he finally did, but without success. When he was asked who the other conspirators were he of course could not name any. He was a Christian. While he was in the USA getting his PhD he married an American. She was the one who later persuaded Tu and her family to return to China because the situation there had supposedly gotten much better (under Mao). Tu and her family returned to China by ship via Europe. Instead of their motor car they took a used piano with them. Then came the Cultural Revolution and everything was taken away from Tu, including two Bibles, all photographs, all phonograph records, and all books because they were "capitalistic". Tu was sent out to the country to work as a farm labourer and later she was employed as a laboratory assistant. At the time of our visit she was the deputy doctor at the Institute of Pathology in Shanghai. Gu was head of the national lymphoma research programme, which was centrally organized. Tu was able to study virtually all cases of lymphoma in China. There was no special equipment, however, not even a typewriter (because of the complicated Chinese characters), just a huge device for documents.

On 9 May I held the first part of a lymph node seminar at the military academy. There were 250 eager listeners, many of whom wore uniforms. After a simple lunch Tu took us to the botanical garden. In the evening we went to the theatre.

The second part of the lymph node seminar was held in the morning of 10 May. The participants expressed their gratitude by sending us on an excursion in the afternoon to Hangzou by train. We were accompanied by Zhang. We were seated in the only carriage with padded seats. The rest of the train was very primitive. The other passengers in the carriage included a soldier and his wife and a Chinese professor of agriculture. The latter explained a plant to us in English and told us about a visit to Germany.

In Hangzou we stayed at what was supposedly the most beautiful hotel in China. The building was old and splendid and the rooms were very large, but it was very hot. Instead of air conditioning there was plenty of green tea. Hangzou lies on the lake where the summer residence of Mao Tse-tung was also located. The next afternoon we retured to Shanghai. There was an American tour group on the train. One of them spoke German with us because he originally came from Koblenz. A Hungarian mathematician told us that he would visit Austria but never Germany. The Americans had been shielded from the Chinese and thus understood very little. A Canadian woman and I had an interesting discussion about the present situation in China and freedom. We also enjoyed conversations with Zhang, who thought that Tu should have a secretary to help her be better organized.

On our last day, 12 May, I discussed T-cell lymphomas and the classification of NHL with Tu. We also spoke about the Chinese working classification, which would be improved later. Tu was very open to the Kiel classification, but she had not yet established a clear standpoint. She was also not well. It was difficult for me to evaluate the situation. Xu and Tu wanted me to become the leader of the Chinese lymphoma group. Xu expressed interest in exchange with Kiel. German colleagues could come to Shanghai for training and Chinese colleagues could go to Kiel. It might be possible to obtain study grants from German foundations.

In my diary I noted that Rappaport and Jaffe had both been in China and had given lectures on the Working Formulation. Lukes had been in Beijing, evidently for more than just a lecture. My influence was more in Shanghai. Even though Zhang had spent two years training at the NCI and had become familiar with the immunohistochemistry of malignant lymphomas, Tu considered Kiel to be the "Mecca". She thought that the Kiel classification was more logical than the Lukes-Collins classification, but her group used "cleaved" instead of centrocytic for linguistic reasons.

Xu organized an elegant farewell lunch at the hotel. Then Tu and I finished our discussion of the Chinese lymphoma classification. I insisted on many changes. In particular I was opposed to distinguishing follicular versus diffuse lymphomas. Tu agreed to make the changes. Later (1987) Xu came to the Lymph Node Registry in Kiel. After my retirement he sent an assistant to work with my former co-worker Feller in Lübeck, Germany. Feller was also invited to Shanghai. I do not know much more about further German-Chinese contacts.

In the afternoon we went into the city to buy presents. At the airport Xu was waiting for us with a special "distinguished guests" document that allowed us to board the Japanese aeroplane quickly. We noticed that there were lots of police at the large terminal, but they were not unfriendly.

2.16.18.3 JAPAN, 12–19 MAY 1984

When we arrived in Tokyo late in the evening Nagai, his daughter, and Suchi were waiting for us at the airport. The next morning Suchi joined us for breakfast. Then Nagai and his daughter accompanied us by aeroplane to Aori, where we were met by Nagai's wife and driven to **Hirosaki**. There we had an interesting conversation with Nagai's wife about the German language, which she thought was more exact and more logical than Japanese. Both Nagai and his head assistant Y. Kamata spoke German. Nagai taught German at the University of Hirosaki.

On 14 May I held a lecture on lymphomas for medical students. The lecture hall was not full, but the listeners were very interested in immunohistochemistry. Nagai had a small department with eight assistants, one of whom was a woman. Kamata owned copies of both the large handbook and the small lymphoma book, both of which he asked me to sign.

On 15 May we travelled by aeroplane and train to **Nagoya**. SUCHI and his wife SIGEKO met us there. The next morning I met with SUCHI and KIKUCHI to discuss T-cell lymphomas. In the afternoon KOJIMA and I met briefly to discuss preparations for the upcoming German-Japanese meeting in Kiel (see p. 96). That afternoon we were invited to a reception for the top members of the Reticuloendothelial Society in Japan.

In his introductory remarks at the **Congress of the Reticuloendothelial Society** on 17 May SUCHI mentioned that that day marked the 10th anniversary of the Kiel classification. I had been invited as the main speaker at the Congress and was treated with special respect. The topic of my lecture was "Malignant Histiocytosis and Related Disorders" (co-authored by FELLER and RADZUN). There were 300–500 listeners. S. WATANABE and NANBA participated in the discussion.

Afterwards we had lunch with Japanese colleagues who had worked with me in Kiel (SATODATE, Y. SUGIJAMA, TASHIRO, EZUMI, KAMIYAMA, M. MOTOI, MORI). We were entertained by E. ISHIKAWA. At the evening reception I was asked to give a speech, in which I praised my Japanese co-workers NAGAI, MORI, and MOHRI. Then I had to answer innumerable questions and hardly had time to eat. AKAZAKI opened a barrel of sake like a beer barrel at the Oktoberfest and we drank the sake out of square wooden cups.

On the second day of the congress I visited the Springer Verlag stand and gave away all the Japanese translations of the little book I had written in collaboration with STEIN. In the evening we had dinner with the "lymphomaniacs" (AKAZAKI, SATO, and others).

On 19 May we left Japan. It was a long trip via Alaska home to Germany.

In retrospect I wrote the following comments in my diary. AKAZAKI was 81 years old and seemed both physically and mentally fit even though he had had tuberculosis. Together with ROBB-SMITH he had been one of the last pupils of ASCHOFF. The year before he had visited Germany with a YMCA group, of which his Christian wife was a member. He had been in the USA only once, 10 years previously. He was very much in tune with Germany. Unfortunately, he did not have a good relationship with the late S. AMANO (professor in Kyoto), who also thought much of German pathology.

SUCHI had spent five years in the USA and got married there. He was born near Nagoya and was originally a physiologist. He was a faithful supporter of the Kiel classification and a very resolute person, even though he was slight in apperance.

In general we gained a lot of ground in Japan. There were still several pro-USA, anti-Germany people, however, including NANBA and several colleagues at the Cancer Institute in Tokyo. IIJIMA would be succeeded by HARA; both of them had worked with F. BÜCHNER in Freiburg. The influence of ASCHOFF was still noticeable. Probably the best Japanese pathologists had been in Freiburg.

2.16.18.4 SIENA, ITALY, 24–26 MAY 1984

At a symposium on **Cytobiology of Leukemias and Lymphomas** I gave a presentation entitled "Morphology and Immunohistology of T Cell Lymphomas" (co-author: FELLER). The main subjects of the presentation were lymphoepithelioid lymphoma (Lennert's lymphoma) and lymphohistiocytic lymphoma. There was a lively discussion with GALTON about "L.B. disease" (lymphohistiocytic lymphoma); "L. B." was one of his patients. GALTON thought the disease was benign. H. VAN DEN BERGHE (geneticist from Louvain, Belgium) said that the demonstration of chromosomal anomalies in one of our cases was not proof of malignancy because his own father had shown such an anomaly in the bone marrow that disappeared spontaneously.

2.16.18.5 KIEL, 24–27 JUNE 1984

The topic of the **Third Japanese-German Workshop on Cancer Research** was "Malignant Lymphomas and Related Disorders". The members of the scientific programme committee were KOJIMA, K. MUNK, and myself. For the German participants the most significant lectures were given by TAKATSUKI and KOJIMA. TAKATSUKI, who had been the first to describe ATLL, reported on clinical and virological studies of ATLL [83,88]. For discussion KOJIMA presented excellent histopathological slides, which he described as "plasma cell dyscrasia with polyneuropathy and endocrine disturbances" and which he distinguished from multiple myeloma. This syndrome is evidently identical with the POEM syndrome described elsewhere in the literature [89].

2.16.18.6 BUENOS AIRES, ARGENTINA, 2–4 SEPTEMBER 1984

At the airport my wife and I were met by BESUSCHIO's wife and daughter, whom we had met when they came to Kiel. We attended the opening ceremony of the **XI. Congress of the International Society of Haematology**, which was held at the *Centro cultural General San Martin*. The lecture halls were nice and the congress was well organized, but when the plenary lectures began there were no slide projectors and this caused a delay. That evening I had conversations with DIEBOLD, GOOD, and others.

On 3 September BESUSCHIO met us at the hotel very early because there was a general strike in progress and there were very few taxis. BESUSCHIO took us to his institute, where we were greeted warmly and met all of his assistants.

The topic of the first symposium at the congress was the pathohistology of the bone marrow. It was moderated by R. Burckhardt. The participants included A. Georgii and Diebold. I was asked to report on mastocytosis; the audience was very interested. Afterwards E.C. Zaino invited me to New York; he was a supporter of the Kiel classification.

In the afternoon the second symposium was moderated by Diebold. I gave a presentation on prelymphomas (myoepithelial sialadenitis, etc.). There were also talks by M. Reynes, Georgii, and Schwarze.

On 4 September I gave a plenary lecture entitled "New Data on Morphology and Immunohistochemistry of T-Cell Lymphomas". Before the session I had an informal, inconclusive conversation with van den Berghe, who gave one of the lectures before mine; his topic was cytogenetics and haematology. J.W. Adamson (from Seattle) gave an excellent lecture on stem cell problems. E. Polli was chairman of the session and introduced me kindly, even mentioning my musical ambitions. Since I felt uneasy I was not able to speak fluently. There was no light where I was standing in front of the slide screen (which was not visible from the rostrum). I had chosen colour transparencies of resin embedded sections, which were of high quality; but I could not make any pithy statements because it was not yet possible to present a definitive concept of T-cell lymphomas. Pure morphology was above the heads of the audience (at least 500). Nevertheless, the listeners were impressed by the transparencies. Afterwards Dorothea Zucker-Franklin asked me if I would give her some photographs for her book. Adamson offered to publish my photographs in »Blood«, of which he was head editor. Later I did not follow up on this offer because the problem of T-cell lymphomas still did not seem to have been solved. Besuschio thanked me for mentioning him and the Argentinean pathologists in my introduction; my praise was important to them politically.

In the afternoon Marina Narbitz took us on a tour of the city. The next day Besuschio drove us to the airport.

2.16.18.7 USA, 5–22 SEPTEMBER 1984

From Buenos Aires we flew via Miami, FL and New York to **Baltimore, MD**. There we were met by D. Mereny, an old friend whom I had met while I was in Erlangen, Germany. He showed us John Hopkins Hospital, where Dorothy Reed had masterfully demonstrated the giant cells of Hodgkin's disease. Risa Mann was now responsible for haematopathology there.

Then we continued on to **Nashville, TN** to visit Collins at Vanderbilt University. I gave a lecture on "Pathology of Mast Cells".

On 14 September we finally reached **San Diego, CA**, where we were welcomed by Lukes and his wife. Lukes was retired, but still worked one or two days per week at the cancer institute in La Jolla, CA, where he examined cases sent for consultation and continued his research. He was annoyed because the third tutorial that had been planned for him in Europe was cancelled because of a meeting in Lugano, Switzerland.

On 16 September we arrived in **Chicago**. I had been invited by Northwestern University to give a lecture. VARIAKOJIS and her husband met us at the airport. The next morning she introduced me to the head of her department, D. G. SCARPELLI, who originally came from Italy. VARIAKOJIS had escaped from Lithuania. The topic of my lecture was T-cell lymphomas. SCARPELLI introduced me; he mentioned that I had been criticizing the histological techniques used in the USA. There was a lively discussion about T-cell lymphomas. MOLNAR was in the audience and enthusiastically expressed her support. Afterwards I was asked to sign many copies of the recent book on lymphomas.

On 19 September we flew back to **Rochester, MN**. BANKS was waiting for us and we spent the evening with him, KADIN, and WARNKE. The next day a **Workshop on Controversies in Lymphoid Pathology** was held at the Mayo Clinic. It was moderated by BANKS, who began by giving a review of current lymphoma research. He was overly enthusiastic about the work of the group in Kiel and maintained that we had been the first to do everything. He said that RAPPAPORT's work was out of date and that LUKES' concepts had become of minor interest. The Working Formulation was not mentioned at all.

During the workshop the following topics were covered and then at the end the participants were expected to take a post-test: immunological methods, classification of B-cell lymphomas (WARNKE); specific categories of lymphoid hyperplasia (FRIZZERA); histiocytic proliferations, Hodgkin's disease (KADIN); differential diagnosis of low-grade neoplasia versus hyperplasia (BANKS); "premalignant" or precursor states of lymphoid hyperplasia (the author); cytochemical methods (LI). There were also several case discussions. In the evening I held the "keynote lecture" on T-cell lymphomas. In his amusing introduction BANKS showed photographs of the Institute of Pathology in Kiel in comparison with the town of Kiel in Wisconsin.

On 21 September there was a discussion with the faculty. I emphasized the importance of optimum techniques and the use of haematological stainings (e.g. Giemsa) before doing immunological analyses. WARNKE asked the participants for special applause in recognition of the Giemsa stained slides that I had shown in my lecture.

In the afternoon I met with G. W. DEWALD, a cytogeneticist. He was very well organized and had analyzed 29 lymph nodes in the past few years. He did not think it was necessary to use the cytogenetic technique of E. J. YUNIS, since he had done comparisons in a blind study. He told me that Gödde-Salz (Kiel) was welcome to visit him.

Banks accompanied us to the airport on 22 September. He admitted that he used the Working Formulation but added the terms of the Kiel classification in parentheses. He complained that there was less scientific freedom in the USA than in Germany. The Working Formulation would prevail in the USA because of the omnipotence of the NCI.

2.16.18.8 UK, 18–21 NOVEMBER 1984

At the invitation of the medical faculty I had a brief **guest professorship** at the University of **Birmingham**. L. Jones and his wife met me at the airport on 18 November and brought me to the elegant home of R. Curran, who had kindly invited me to stay with him. Curran was a highly regarded British scientist and had been president of the Royal College of Pathologists for three years.

On 19 November I visited Jones at the Institute of Pathology. Then I went to see MacLennan, who had just learned of the tragic death of his friend Ford in Australia. We had a candid discussion of several topics, including marginal zone cells; we were joined by a few of his assistants.

At noon there was a reception where I met the dean and many members of the faculty. In the afternoon I gave a lecture on prelymphomas (progressively transformed germinal centres and Sjögren's syndrome). There were relatively few listeners, but the discussion was lively and friendly. Afterwards I attended a faculty meeting, where I was greeted cordially. There were about 50 people at the meeting, including 10 students. The topics of discussion were common faculty matters, in which I did not participate. In the evening Jones invited me to his home outside of Birmingham for dinner.

On 20 November I visited M. J. Owen, an anatomist who was an expert on T-cells. We had a very interesting discussion about the maturation of T-cells in the thymus. He said that interdigitating cells are responsible for the maturation. He also told me about experiments concerning the rearrangement of T-cell genes.

Afterwards I visited the department of radiology. There were no facilities for lymphangiography. Thus staging was not possible and many cases of NHL were probably overtreated.

In the late morning I held a lecture on NHL. MacLennan mentioned in the discussion that the Kiel classification had now been fully confirmed immunologically. Later in the afternoon I gave another lecture on the pathology of T-cell lymphomas. There were about 250 listeners, including many students. The dean made introductory remarks. I was able to speak freely and the lecture went well.

That evening I was invited to dinner with about 15 members of the faculty at the staff house of the University. I sat between the dean and CURRAN, both of whom paid me complements in their speeches. I was flattered by many who praised my English. At his home afterwards CURRAN gave me a lesson about the various kinds of whisky. During my whole stay in Birmingham he took especially good care of me, for which I was very grateful.

On 21 November CURRAN and JONES and their wives accompanied me to **Woodstock**. I thought this was very kind of them because they were very busy. We drove through beautiful autumn countryside and saw the village where SHAKESPEARE had lived. After an early lunch in Woodstock we went to visit ROBB-SMITH. He was very glad to see us, even though he was not well and his vision had become very poor. In spite of his poor health he was working on a book about the faculty of Oxford University in the 19th century. He was up to date on lymphoma research and still a staunch supporter of the Kiel classification. He thought this was the only classification that was of proven clinical relevance and still simple to use and reproducible. His wife was very kind and cheery. She took care of him at home in Woodstock until he died on 2 January 2000.

In the afternoon MASON met me and drove me to his laboratory. I asked him whether it had the capacity to do DNA analyses of the cases of T-cell lymphoma collected in Kiel. He agreed.

2.16.19 1985

The diagnosis and manifestation of T-cell lymphomas continued to be of great interest in 1985. One of the most important findings was the demonstration of the clonal rearrangement of the T-cell receptor β-chain gene by MASON's research group [68] and by H. GRIESSER at the laboratory of T. W. MAK and in Kiel [69,90].

2.16.19.1 PUERTO DE LA CRUZ, TENERIFE, 8–10 MARCH 1985

The ***I. Reunion de Patología Canaria*** was organized by OLGA FERRER-ROCA of the *Universidad de la Laguna*. The topic of the meeting was the pathology of lymphomas on the Canary Islands. The participants were pathologists from the Canary Islands and Spain. I was invited to hold a lecture on the prognostic and diagnostic value of the Kiel classification of NHL and to give the introduction to a seminar on malignant lymphomas, which was held by SCHWARZE. He also gave a lecture on extranodal NHL. FERRER-ROCA used to work in Barcelona, Spain, had spent four weeks in Kiel in 1981, and was now director of the new Institute of Pathology at the University. After my presentations there were several lectures on malignant lymphomas on the Canary Islands and in Barcelona. Immunohistochemical and clinical data were emphasized.

2.16.19.2 KIEL, 24–30 APRIL 1985

SUCHI came to Kiel to work with us on T-cell lymphomas. Together we sat at the microscope and studied about 200 cases, most of which I had discussed with TU (see p. 87) and with experts on HTLV-positive ATLL from Japan (KIKUCHI and SATO [86]). Our observations were combined with histochemical findings (presented by FELLER) and cytogenetic data (presented by GÖDDE-SALZ). The result was a new classification of T-cell lymphomas that was published by SUCHI et al. [91].

2.16.19.3 STOCKHOLM, SWEDEN, 6 JUNE 1985

At a meeting of Scandinavian pathologists I gave a lecture on "Borderline Problems of Hodgkin's and Non-Hodgkin's Lymphomas". BIBERFELD invited DORFMAN and me to attend. At the end of my presentation I said that the borderline between Hodgkin's disease and NHL is not sharp because there is neither a specific cell type (Sternberg-Reed cells) nor a specific immunological marker (Ki-1) that proves or excludes Hodgkin's disease. Hence we shall have to look for more specific markers and use other techniques, e.g. gene rearrangement analyses, in order to learn whether or not Hodgkin's disease and NHL overlap.

2.16.19.4 KIEL, 10–11 JUNE 1985

MACLENNAN accepted an invitation to Kiel and held two lectures. His visit was very stimulating. We discussed the various types of cells in lymphoid tissue and found that we agreed on all important points.

2.16.19.5 PRAGUE, CZECHOSLOVAKIA, 3–6 SEPTEMBER 1985

The topic of the **International Symposium of the UICC** was "Recent Approaches to Chronic Lymphoproliferative Diseases". MATHÉ gave an introduction entitled "Integrating Positition of Electron Microscopy in Diagnosis of Malignant Lymphomas". The title of my main lecture was "Morphology and Immunohistochemistry of T-Cell Lymphomas. New Results". I also gave a talk on "Lymphoepithelioid Lymphoma. Pathology and Differential Diagnosis". B. BEDNÁŘ was critical of this entity.

2.16.19.6 KIEL, 13–15 SEPTEMBER 1985

The **Second Dermatohistopathology Meeting** was held under the auspices of the International Society of Dermatohistopathology and organized by E. CHRISTOPHERS. On 14 September I held a special lecture entitled "Malignant Histiocytosis and Related Disorders". ZUCKER-FRANKLIN gave a comprehensive presentation on "Phylogeny and Structure of the Granulocytes". She also visited us at the Institute of Pathology, and we had a good conversation about various problems.

2.16.19.7 ATHENS, 4–5 OCTOBER 1985

PAPACHARALAMPOUS invited me to give a lecture entitled "Malignant Histiocytoses and Related Neoplasias" for pathologists and haematologists. It was held in a lecture hall at the military hospital, where General TINIAKOS was the director and professor of pathology. He greeted me heartily in German, for which I thanked him when I began my presentation in German. I said that the fate of the German language was similar to that of Old Greek, since both languages had been largely dismantled but were still essential for understanding ancient and modern philosophy. Then I continued my presentation in English. In retrospect I was somewhat disappointed because I should have spoken about the Kiel classification instead of histiocytosis. I acquiesced to my hosts' request, however, since I and others had misjudged the current state of lymphoma classification in Greece.

After the lecture I enjoyed meeting and speaking with many people, including E. PATSOURIS and C. H. KITTAS. RAPPAPORT had been in Greece awhile ago and had presented his revised classification.

In my diary I noted that PANGALIS was favourable to Rappaport. PATSOURIS would probably have a difficult time because he was an emphatic supporter of the Kiel classification, but he would probably prevail. KITTAS evidently gave the clinicians diagnoses according to the Rappaport classification and the Working Formulation; but he denied this to me.

In Greece those who studied and diagnosed lymphomas seemed to waver between the Kiel classification and the American classifications. About half of them were oriented towards the USA. ANAGNOSTOU had spent a year working with Lukes. Pangalis had worked with Rappaport for two years. Papacharalampous had studied in Germany (with H. Meessen) and was a supporter of German pathology, but he was not very forceful. His students Papadimitriou (spent 18 months in Kiel) and Patsouris (spent three years in Kiel) would have to fight. They had done good work. The influence of Rappaport and the clinicians who had studied in the USA was very strong. During my visit Anagnostou appeared to be changing her mind and offered to come to Kiel to help me revise the book on reactive lymphadenopathy. (This never took place. Instead a CD-ROM on reactive and inflammatory lymphadenopathy was produced together with Diebold.)

2.16.19.8 VIENNA, 6–9 OCTOBER 1985

At the annual meeting of the **Austrian and German Societies of Haematology and Oncology** I gave a lecture on T-cell lymphomas (*"Zur Immunhistochemie und Morphologie der T-Zell-Lymphome"*; co-authored by Feller).

2.16.20 ATTEMPTS TO FORM A EUROPEAN-AMERICAN ALLIANCE, 1986

2.16.20.1 KIEL, 26–28 JANUARY 1986

At a meeting of the ELC one of the topics was preparing for the negotiations at the later meeting in New Orleans, LA, USA (see below).

Two weeks later I met with Brittinger in Frankfurt a. M. to talk about clinical aspects in preparation for the negotiations in New Orleans.

2.16.20.2 NEW ORLEANS, LA, USA, 8–12 MARCH 1986

Banks was the only person who knew about my arrival in New Orleans as a "surprise guest". Since he was a member of the board of the **Society for Hematopathology** I asked him to present my proposal concerning the inclusion of European haematopathologists as a separate division of the Society ("European Division"). He agreed to do so at the board meeting on 8 March.

In the morning of 9 March I had breakfast with Banks, Dorfman, and Frizzera. Then Banks and I went for a walk in the French Quarter and along the Mississippi River. He told me about the board meeting and was very pessimistic about adding a European section to the Society. Later I inferred from a conversation with Kadin and his wife that Kadin had proposed me for membership on the board. He was discouraged that his proposal had been rejected. I also had a conversation with DORFMAN, even though he had just given up his position on the board of the Society. "As a South African" he was in favour of international cooperation, but he said that he no longer had any influence in the Society. His comment was: "What would happen if the Japanese and South Americans came to the Society with the same request?" I realized from this and other comments that the wind was blowing in the wrong direction and gave up my intention of presenting my proposal at the general meeting of the Society.

Before the meeting I had an opportunity to speak with RAPPAPORT. He was president of the Society and said that he would support all of my proposals. He asked me to put the European requests into writing and to send him copies of my previous correspondence with BERARD.

The **Annual Meeting of the Society for Hematopathology** was held in the afternoon of 9 March. There were four presentations announced as "A Potpourri of Hematopathology". The topics were: classification of leukaemia (J.H. BECKSTEAD), immunotyping of lymphoma (R.R. TUBBS), cutaneous lymphoid infiltrates (BANKS), and histiocytic syndromes (L.P. DEHNER). BANKS' presentation was enjoyable because he had a good sense of humour.

This was followed by a business meeting. DORFMAN diplomatically greeted all of the participants from overseas (including I. KATAYAMA, RILKE, and myself). He referred to the European problem in just one sentence.

Afterwards BANKS organized a dinner at a very good French restaurant. I enjoyed the evening with HARRIS, VARIAKOJIS, C. KJELDSBERG, FRIZZERA, and BANKS. HARRIS had just been appointed as head of the programme committee and wanted to invite some Europeans to a meeting to discuss Hodgkin's disease. She asked me about the reasons for my proposal. KJELDSBERG had worked with RAPPAPORT six years ago. He originally came from Norway and now lived in Utah. He expressed interest in a sabbatical in Kiel (unfortunately, this never came about).

A meeting of the **US-Canadian Division of the International Academy of Pathology** [92] began on 10 March. I had lunch with COLLINS and his wife, who were pleasantly surprised that I was there. BRUNNING also joined us. He asked me to say something about a case of Ki-1-positive lymphoma during the slide seminar in the evening. The afternoon session on haematopathology included presentations on the following topics: Castleman's disease, monocytoid B-cell lymphoma, malignant lymphoma in X-linked lymphoproliferative syndrome, and angiotropic (intravascular) large cell lymphoma.

In the morning of 11 March there were five good presentations. The topics included mediastinal large cell lymphoma, lymphomatoid granulomatosis, angiocentric lymphoma, and AILD. The authors of the latter presentation mentioned "key papers" by FRIZZERA, LUKES, NATHWANI, and SHIMOYAMA but none by the research group in Kiel (H. KNECHT [26,27]). They distinguished AILD from AILD-type T-cell lymphoma. They found T-cell receptor gene rearrangements in two cases of AILD and in five cases of AILD T-cell lymphoma. I presented the data obtained by GRIESSER (at the laboratory of MAK) and these were acknowledged by the audience. In the ensuing discussion H. A. AZAR pointed out to the chairperson that I was Professor LENNERT from Germany and that I should have been officially introduced. During the break I thanked him for this kind gesture.

After the morning session a business meeting was held by Raven Press; the moderator was STERNBERG. I sat together with SLAVIN, AZAR, and colleagues from Winston Salem, NC. In the afternoon there were two presentations that put me into an embarrassing situation. HSU thought that I had said that Sternberg-Reed cells were interdigitating reticulum cells. R. S. NEIMAN asked me to comment, but I left the matter open so as not to discredit HSU. GATTER presented a paper on paragranuloma, which kindled a lively discussion between him and DORFMAN and NEIMAN. I came to GATTER's defense, which probably helped to re-establish a good relationship between me and MASON's research group.

A long course entited "Malignant Lymphoma, Leukemia and the Immune System: From Cacophony to Clarity" was held on 12 March. It was directed by BERARD and DORFMAN. The only paper by the research group in Kiel mentioned by DORFMAN [93] in his introduction was the one about follicular lymphoma that I had presented in Nagoya 1973. In the published version of his remarks DORFMAN also cited the lecture that I gave in Zurich (in 1966!) on the European concept of lymphoma classification.

NATHWANI [94] gave a lecture on the classification of NHL. He said that it was necessary to improve the Working Formulation and mentioned numerous suggestions. These included adding a category for immunocytoma and an "intermediate" category (equivalent to centrocytic lymphoma). Three of the existing categories should be divided: "mixed cell" into B-cell and T-cell types, "large cell" into cleaved and non-cleaved types, and "immunoblastic" into B plasmacytoid and T-cell types. Additional terms for the classification of peripheral T-cell lymphomas were also necessary, including categories for ATLL, AILD, and angiocentric lymphoma. NATHWANI then presented a modified Working Formulation. He cited only two findings by the research group in Kiel (pseudofollicular structures in chronic lymphocytic leukaemia and another that I did not take note of) and did not mention the Kiel classification as a separate classification. At least he understood that immunocytoma was an entity. In his mind the Working Formulation was the only valid classification. I thought that his presentation was confusing.

WARNKE gave a lecture on "B-Cell Lymphomas and Related Disorders in Immunologic Perspective". The only findings of the research group in Kiel that he cited were the Ki-67 data and he did not mention STEIN at all. J. COSSMAN spoke about Hodgkin's disease, T-cell neoplasms, and related disorders. He mentioned the Ki-1 problem, but did not say anything about the Ki-1 antibody. His research group had their own equivalent antibody.

There were many more lectures that day, but I did not hear all of them because I had to leave at noon.

During the meeting many people asked me why I had come (e.g. DORFMAN and RAPPAPORT). I answered somewhat sarcastically that I had come to meet "clarity". COLLINS was annoyed over the title of the course and intended to write a letter to the president. He scribbled on my programme: "In a world of blind men the one-eyed man is king". My surprise appearance at the meeting troubled NATHWANI, who said that my attendance was unnecessary since I already knew everything.

Later, when I spoke with KADIN he told me that he thought my presence at the meeting was a good idea and he hoped that there would be cooperation between the USA and Europe. BRUNNING was of the same opinion. RADASZKIEWICZ was shocked that Europe and Kiel did not seem to exist for the Americans. An Iranian whom I met at the hotel told me that it was an insult that my excellent book had not been mentioned at all. When I spoke with HARRIS I said that I was discouraged because my proposal had been turned down so bluntly. She was very optimistic and thought that in 10 years the whole world would be speaking the Kiel language.

In retrospect I noted in my diary that the surprise "coup" had been a success because it put the Europeans and Kiel in the spotlight. The intrigues incited by influential people had been disturbed. It had become obvious that some Americans intended to isolate the Europeans. On the other hand, there were many colleagues who were familiar with books by the Kiel research group and who greeted me enthusiastically.

2.16.20.3 AFTER-EFFECTS, APRIL 1986

Several American lymphoma experts spoke with the President-elect of the Society for Hematopathology, BRUNNING, who suggested that they write him a letter. In the letter they stated that they supported my attendance at the meetings in New Orleans and also my proposal concerning cooperation between the USA and Europe. They suggested that meetings be organized in the USA to discuss cases for which detailed clinical information and immunological data were available (similar to the regular meetings of the European

Lymphoma Study Group). Evidently BRUNNING's reaction to the letter was positive, but I do not know any further details.

On 17 April I sent a letter to RAPPAPORT, then president of the Society for Hematopathology. I wrote him the following:

"After returning from ... [New Orleans] ... and having conversations with several European colleagues concerning the discussions that took place in New Orleans, I want to explain to you our standpoint. First, though, I must take the precaution of saying that this standpoint must still be approved by the members of the European Lymphoma Study Group at its next meeting in October.

"Following the discussions in New Orleans we think that at the present time it would be better for our group – which includes about 120 members from practically every country of Europe – to offer to become a Section for Hematopathology in the European Society of Pathology. The European Society of Pathology [LLOMBART-BOSCH] was enthusiastic in its response to our inquiry whether they would accept us as a Section for Hematopathology and offered us complete freedom to hold our meetings separately or jointly with them. By no means does this rule out joint meetings with the Society for Hematopathology.

"We could, with complete autonomy, hold joint meetings with our American colleagues in the Society for Hematopathology. We propose biennial joint meetings to be held alternately in the USA and Europe. [...] At these meetings we could develop a scientific program and hear reports from both continents. This would certainly contribute to further scientific progress. – The workshops carried out by us would take place at the conclusion of the scientific program. Naturally it would be impossible for all members from both continents to take part. A workshop with more than 100 participants and cases would certainly not be practicable. We already have somewhat more than 100 applicants to our next European workshop. Only those who can contribute an immunohistochemically investigated case are being accepted, so that about 100 cases may be discussed at the workshop. – Joint meetings involving participants from both continents must be so organized as to enable an adequate number of participants from each continent without becoming impracticable. – This proposal does not rule out that we Europeans can also collaborate actively within the Society for Hematopathology. In fact, about 20 Europeans are paying members of the Society, most of whom appear in the list of addresses I made available to COSTAN BERARD [in my letter of 23 December 1980].

"It would please me very much if the Society for Hematopathology responds favorably to our proposal. I am very grateful to you for wanting to contribute so positively to this end."

In the discussions I had had in New Orleans with Rappaport and other members of the board of the Society for Hematopathology I pointed out that the original plan of Berard, Dorfman, and myself was for it to be an *international* society and that I was supposed to be a founding member representing the European side. Berard had been in favour of this proposal and had suggested in his letter of 23 December 1980 naming the society "The International Society of Hematopathology". Hence I sent Rappaport excerpts from my correspondence with Berard and added some timely comments.

2.16.20.4 FOUNDING OF THE SOCIETY FOR HEMATOPATHOLOGY IN RETROSPECT

The Society was officially founded on **1 September 1981**. I did not find out until later that I was one of the founding members when I received a document. The first annual meeting was held on 28 February 1982 in Boston in the form of a symposium on T-cell lymphomas. Dorfman was chairman of the meeting and Berard moderated the business meeting. Unfortunately, I was not able to be there because I had already agreed to attend the UCLA symposium that was being held at the same time (see p. 75).

In his letter of 30 November 1981 Berard wrote me the following: "I would also appreciate your advice about how we might proceed in Europe. You once said that you would consider being an officer of the Society. Would you be willing to organize and serve as founding President of the European (or German?) division of the Society for Hematopathology? By April, when Ron [Dorfman] visits you, we should have both experience from the First Annual Meeting and a definite idea of what will be possible at the Sydney Congress of the I.A.P. Ron and I both greatly appreciate and value your advice and active participation in plans from now into the future."

On 22 December 1981 I wrote Berard an answer and sent a copy to Dorfman. In it I said: "I think it would be the best to discuss the whole problem while Ron is here in Kiel in April. Then we will have time to consider each question carefully."

Unfortunately, the discussion with Dorfman never took place because he did not come to Kiel. There was no further correspondence. According to a letter that Berard wrote to Rappaport on 8 July 1986, however, Berard explained why he had dropped the plans to form an international society: he "learned that founding an international society would be clearly beyond our capabilities with regard to legal, fiscal, and logistic considerations." After considering an association with a number of other existing societies, Berard suggested that German haematopathologists form an organization within the German division of the International Academy of Pathology and that I should get in contact with the president of the German division, GEDIGK, "to set up a Society for Hematopathology affiliated with this division. [BERARD] would be pleased if every division of the IAP would eventually have a Society for Hematopathology. If enough divisions were to do so, then we could consider banding together as the International Society for Hematopathology..." Finally, BERARD suggested that the matter be discussed "face-to-face" with DORFMAN, RAPPAPORT, and myself at the next congress of the International Academy of Pathology in Vienna (31 August – 5 September 1986, see below) in order to "clear the air". Such a conversation never took place.

2.16.21 FURTHER EVENTS, 1986–1987

2.16.21.1 APRIL–JULY 1986

Three clinical-theoretical meetings took place in **Deidesheim** (Germany), **Würzburg** (Germany), and **Basel** (Switzerland). Two lectures on T-cell lymphomas were held in France and Norway. SOTTO invited me to speak at **"Assises d'Anatomie pathologique"** in **Grenoble** (3–5 April). DELSOL and DIEBOLD had also been asked to speak. The second opportunity to speak on T-cell lymphomas was in **Oslo** (6–7 May). The lecture was part of a lymph node slide seminar held at the School of Medicine.

2.16.21.2 VIENNA, 27 AUGUST – 5 SEPTEMBER 1986

At the **5th European Conference on Sarcoidosis and Other Granulomatous Disorders**, 27–30 August, I gave a talk on "Epithelioid Cells in Malignant Tumors Including Malignant Lymphomas". I demonstrated two types of epithelioid cell reaction, namely type I (in small clusters) and type II (in large sheets). After discussing these reactions in inflammatory disorders I also presented the findings in lymphoepithelioid lymphoma. At the Conference I met W. JONES WILLIAMS from Wales. He expressed interest in visiting Kiel. He emphasized the secretory function of epithelioid cells, in contrast to the phagocytotic function of macrophages. J. CHURG and H. L. JOACHIM also contributed to the discussion.

Immediately following the Conference, the **XVIth International Congress of the International Academy of Pathology** began on 31 August. At a symposium on "Lymphoma-like Lymphadenopathies" on 3 September I gave a talk on angioimmunoblastic lymphadenopathy and presented the T-cell gene rearrangement data of GRIESSER and the cytogenetic data obtained by

Schlegelberger. Banks commented that we were ahead of the Americans in this field of research. The day before (2 September) Diebold and I had given a slide seminar entitled "Malignant Hodgkin's and Non-Hodgkin's Lymphomas".

2.16.21.3 FAR EAST, 22 SEPTEMBER – 7 OCTOBER 1986

On 22 September I gave a lecture on the pathology of NHL in **Beijing**. At a meeting of Chinese and German physicians in **Wuhan** (25–27 September) I presented the results of the German-Chinese-Japanese study of T-cell lymphomas. The topics of the meeting were very heterogeneous. I gave the same lecture on the pathology of NHL in **Shanghai** (28–29 September). There I enjoyed seeing Xu again.

On 30 September I flew on to **Hong Kong** to visit Faith Ho at her institute. On 1 October I gave a lecture at the old university (University of Hong Kong) entitled "The Kiel Classification of Non-Hodgkin's Lymphomas – Discussion on B-Cell Lymphomas". The lecture hall was full and the atmosphere was very positive. The next day I gave the corresponding lecture "The Kiel Classification of Non-Hodkgin's Lymphomas – Discussion on T-Cell Lymphomas" at the new university (The Chinese University of Hong Kong). My host was J. C. K. Lee. The lecture hall was overcrowded and the atmosphere was excellent. Afterwards Lee gave me a university necktie and invited me to give a main lecture at the meeting of the International Academy of Pathology in 1994. Of course I accepted the invitation.

Next I flew to **Singapore** to visit Ivy Sng. She was the highly respected director of a relatively small institute (10 employees, almost all of whom were women). On 4 October I gave a lecture on NHL. At dinner one evening I met Shanmugaratnam.

2.16.21.4 CHICAGO, 7–12 MARCH 1987

The **Society for Hematopathology** again met in conjunction with the International Academy of Pathology. The topic was "Controversies in Hodgkin's Disease" and it was moderated by Harris and Rappaport. Stein gave a lecture on "Immunologic and Tissue Culture Studies in Hodgkin's Disease" using two slide projectors. My lecture was entitled "Progressive Transformation of Germinal Centers: Clinical Significance and Relationship to Lymphocytic Predominance Hodgkin's Disease. The Kiel Experience". Dorfman spoke on the same topic with respect to the Stanford experience, but did not present any new findings. In his lecture "Clinical Relevance of Morphologic

Studies in Hodgkin's Disease" ROSENBERG concluded that morphology was irrelevant. He said that the treatment for all types of Hodgkin's disease at his hospital was the same. In the discussion I argued that that would mean that the lymphocytic predominance type would be treated with overdoses.

In the evening of 8 March I had dinner with HARRIS, DORFMAN, and a few other colleagues. The atmosphere was pleasant. The next day I joined COLLINS and his wife for dinner.

2.16.21.5 GARDEN CITY, LONG ISLAND, NY, USA, 13–14 MARCH 1987

Together with LIEBERMAN I held a **slide seminar** for the **New York State Society of Pathologists** and the Nassau County Society of Pathologists at the Nassau Academy of Medicine. I had been invited by the president of the State Society, ZAINO, who had heard my lecture in 1984 in Buenos Aires (see p. 96) and had promised to invite me. N.S. TAYLOR (born in Berlin in 1930) acted as my gracious host and made me feel very welcome. LIEBERMAN contributed two of the ten cases discussed in the seminar and also gave a lecture on Langerhans' cell histiocytosis. I held a lecture on the Kiel classification.

After the symposium I exchanged memories with ELIZABETH WU and she gave me a present from her mother (TU) who had died in 1986. While we were having this somewhat sad conversation my suitcase containing about 600 colour transparencies was stolen. The hotel set off an alarm, but nothing was found. Fortunately, LIEBERMAN was there and made sure that the matter would be pursued. F. COLLIER called the Fire Department and the episode was even mentioned on televison.

2.16.21.6 BOSTON, MA, 15–17 MARCH 1987

On 15 March I had to leave for Boston without the colour transparencies. I had been invited to give two lectures there, but these of course had to be cancelled. Instead I improvised at the blackboard for HARRIS, PINKUS, a colleague from Iceland, and several co-workers.

2.16.21.7 OBERHAUSEN, GERMANY, 23 MARCH – 7 APRIL 1987

While I was in the hospital for surgery my secretary informed me that the stolen suitcase had been found by a woman in her yard in the Bronx. The pathologists there were returning it by airmail. I made sure that the woman was rewarded for her kindness.

2.17 FOUNDING OF THE EUROPEAN LYMPHOMA STUDY GROUP

2.17.1 KIEL, 7–8 NOVEMBER 1980

Lymphoma research in Kiel had been generously supported by the DFG since 1973 ("*Sonderforschungsbereich*", see p. 13). During the review process in 1978 the question arose whether our work had been receiving enough international attention. An answer was to be found at a symposium organized by the speaker of the *Sonderforschungsbereich*. The symposium was entitled **"Recent Data from the Characterization of Malignant Lymphoma"** [95]. It was held at the University of Kiel. The international response to the invitation was astonishing. More than 200 people registered for the symposium, almost half of them from outside Germany. Eleven presentations were held by respected scientists from other countries and 15 by researchers from Kiel. The symposium was an overwhelming success. At the end of it Robb-Smith went to the microphone and congratulated the hosts with moving words commending the substance of the symposium and the stimulation it generated. He also proposed that the participating pathologists join forces in order to train in the diagnosis of lymphoma using the criteria of the Kiel classification.

To our great surprise more than 50 pathologists showed up at the Institute of Pathology in the afternoon of 8 November to form a study group that would meet at regular intervals to learn more about lymphoma diagnosis according to the Kiel classification and to exchange experience. Even Robb-Smith, although he was over 80 years old, attended this meeting and was one of the enthusiastic initiators of the study group.

That was how the **European Lymphoma Study Group** (ELSG) came into existence. It was just to consider this group to be an expansion of the ELC and to be the legitimate predecessor of the European Association for Haematopathology.

An interval of two years was chosen for the regular meetings that would take place in different European cities. There were several prerequisites for participation in the meetings. (1) Each participant would have to provide one unstained and one Giemsa-stained section from a case of his/her choice. (2) In addition 15 unstained sections had to be sent to the laboratory in Kiel for special stainings. (3) The clinical data were also to be sent to Kiel for copying and distribution to all the participants. At the meeting each participant would present his own case and the reasons for the diagnosis he had made.

The positive reaction to the symposium encouraged the DFG to continue its generous support of the *Sonderforschungsbereich* in Kiel.

At a meeting of the ELC in London a short time later in November there was much delight and relief over the news from Kiel.

2.17.2 KIEL, 20–24 OCTOBER 1981

The **first workshop of the ELSG** was held at the Institute of Pathology. SCHWARZE was the secretary (Fig. 16). The small microscopy room at the Institute had to accommodate 91 pathologists from 26 different countries (the USA was not included this time). The participants came from West Germany (6), France (6), The Netherlands (6), Belgium (6), Spain (6), Italy (6), Switzerland (6), the UK (6), Sweden (5), Austria (3), Yugoslavia (3), Poland (3), East Germany (3), Denmark (3), Finland (3), Greece (3), Turkey (2), Norway (2), Czechoslovakia (2), Hungary (2), Israel (2), Rumania (2), Portugal (2), Luxembourg (1), Bulgaria (1), and Iceland (1).

All cases were presented on television screens and discussed. Each participant received a set of slides stained with Giemsa. WRIGHT and ISAACSON were sitting in the first row (Fig. 17). ROBB-SMITH was in the second row. It was hardly noticeable how old he was or that he could use only one (glaucomatous) eye. He sat there the whole time and never complained about the hard seats or the fact that his vision became worse during the Workshop (which he admitted to me later). The participants also included MIODUSZEWSKA, NÉZELOF, DIEBOLD, and BÜRKI.

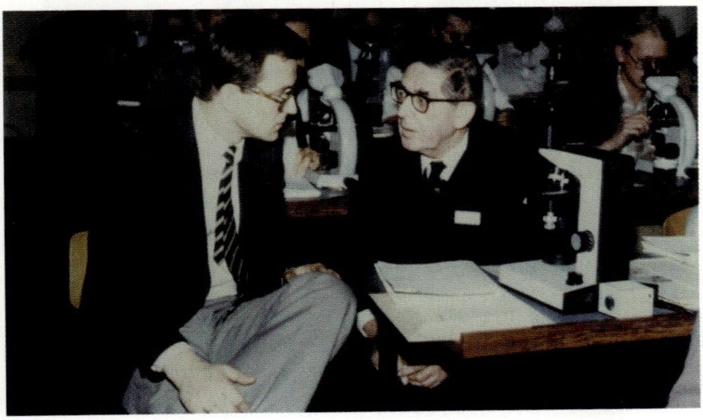

Fig. 16 First workshop of the European Lymphoma Study Group in the microscopy room at the Institute of Pathology in Kiel, Germany, 1981. *Left to right:* E.-W. SCHWARZE (organizer of the workshop), A. H. T. ROBB-SMITH

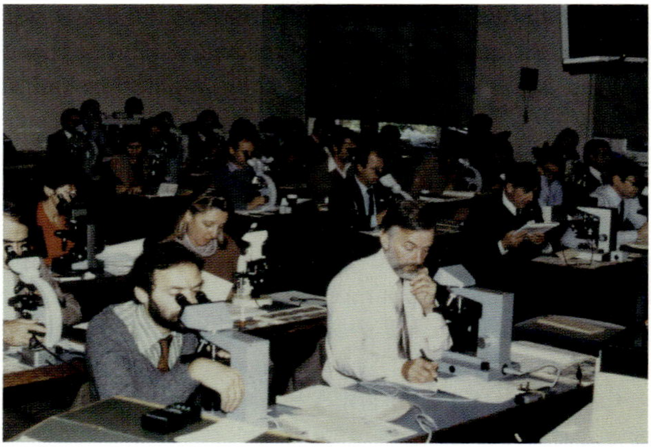

Fig. 17 Same occasion as Fig. 16. *First row:* P. G. ISAACSON, D. H. WRIGHT. *Second row, middle:* ANNE MARIE MANDARD

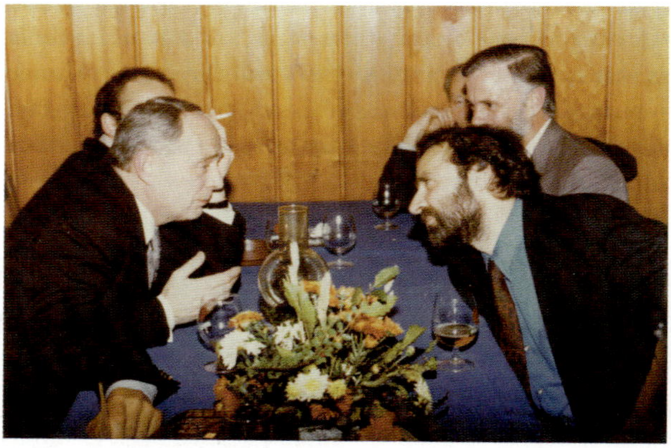

Fig. 18 Same occasion as Fig. 16. Lively discussion at the closing dinner. *Left front:* G. KELÉNYI. *Right front:* P. G. ISAACSON. *Behind:* D. H. WRIGHT

The case discussions were interspersed with lectures. For example, ISAACSON reported on intestinal lymphomas, which he considered to be histiocytic. On Saturday I ended the session early because NOËL's data on Lennert's lymphoma were not convincing enough. In general, the response to the workshop was enthusiastic. ROBB-SMITH gave a very humorous speech at the final dinner (Fig. 18).

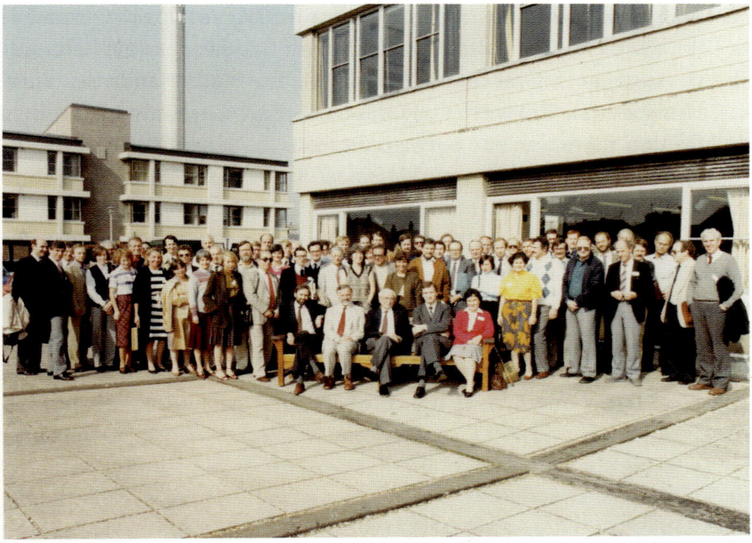

Fig. 19 Second Workshop of the European Lymphoma Study Group in Southampton, UK, 1983. Most of the participants are shown. *First row, sitting, left to right*: P. G. ISAACSON, D.H. WRIGHT, the author, E.-W. SCHWARZE, ANNA TU

2.17.3 SOUTHAMPTON, UK, 25–28 SEPTEMBER 1983

The **second workshop of the ELSG** (Fig. 19) was organized by WRIGHT. At the time STEIN was already in Oxford and helped with the organization. He evidently had little time for me. At least we were able to complete a lymphoma review. WRIGHT did not ask for any help from me. So I was very reserved during the case discussions and even excused myself part of the time in order to prepare my lecture.

On the first day ISAACSON gave a lecture on extranodal lymphomas. My presentation was scheduled for the second day. I reported on the results of the German-Japanese workshop on T-cell lymphomas. TU gave a humorous, stimulating lecture on T-cell lymphomas in China [96]. She had data on more than 9,000 lymphomas. On the third day STEIN and MASON reported on "Advances in the Use of Immunohistochemistry in the Study of Lymphomas".

Case discussions filled the times between the lectures. As at the workshop in Kiel, each participant was required to contribute a case.

The number of participants was somewhat smaller than at the first workshop, but there were a number of auditors from Southampton. The 72 participants came from the following countries: the UK (10), West Germany (9), France (7), Switzerland (7), Italy (7), Denmark (5), Sweden (4), Belgium (4), Spain (4), Austria (3), Greece (2), Poland (2), The Netherlands (2), Yugoslavia (1), Hungary (1), Norway (1), Finland (1), East Germany (1), and China (1). In addition there was one participant from the USA (BANKS).

2.17.4 TOULOUSE, FRANCE, 1–3 APRIL 1985

The **third workshop of the ELSG** was organized by DELSOL. The topics were lymphadenitis, AIDS, Hodgkin's disease, angioimmunoblastic lymphadenopathy, and T-cell lymphomas. There was also a slide seminar dealing mainly with lymphadenitis; it was probably the best slide seminar of the ELSG.

2.17.5 BRUSSELS, 27–29 OCTOBER 1986

R. HEIMANN organized the **fourth workshop of the ELSG**. He had a great sense of humour. This was the first time that not only BANKS but also HARRIS from the USA attended, and they asked to be invited to all the next workshops. They said that they wanted to use the "format" of the ELSG workshops in the USA.

2.17.6 GENEVA, 14–15 MARCH 1988

The **fifth workshop of the ELSG** was integrated into the first meeting of the European Association for Haematopathology (see p. 120). The workshop was organized by SCHWARZE and the main topic was extranodal lymphomas, with special emphasis on those of MALT.

3 FOUNDING OF THE EUROPEAN ASSOCIATION FOR HAEMATOPATHOLOGY

3.1 PRELUDE, 1986–1988

In preparation for the mission in New Orleans there were several gatherings. On 30 April 1986 I met in Kiel with PALLESEN, the designated secretary of a European society.

The members of the ELC gathered in Utrecht, The Netherlands, 18–19 July 1986. Then the ELC met in Brussels, Belgium, on 27 October 1986 to discuss the "draft of the by-laws for a European Society for Haematopathology" that had been prepared by DIEBOLD and WRIGHT.

On 4 November 1986 KAPANÇI wrote me that he had spoken with a lawyer about the possibility of founding a European Society for Haematopathology in Switzerland. The lawyer had agreed, but suggested using a different name (see below).

Further meetings of the ELC to discuss the by-laws and the programme of the first meeting took place in Milan (25–26 February 1987 and 15–16 September 1987) and in Paris (3–5 December 1987).

3.1.1 KIEL, 9–11 DECEMBER 1987

The ELC decided that the main topic of the first meeting should be the pathology of lymphomas of the gastrointestinal tract. Since ISAACSON had first defined MALT lymphoma, I invited him to Kiel to discuss this entity and place it into context with the other gastrointestinal lymphomas. He accepted the invitation and came to Kiel twice. During his second visit we developed a preliminary classification of these lymphomas (Table 2). This draft was later revised and published in 1994 [97].

Table 2 Draft of a preliminary classification of lymphomas of the gastrointestinal tract (worked out together with Isaacson in Kiel in 1987)

B-cell types	
	1. Low-grade malignant B-cell lymphomas of MALT, including immunocytoma
	2. High-grade malignant B-cell lymphomas of MALT (centroblastic, immunoblastic, Burkitt's lymphoma, large cell anaplastic, undefined) with or without evidence of low-grade component
	3. Immunoproliferative small intestinal disease (IPSID; Mediterranean lymphoma)
	4. Centrocytic lymphoma (later renamed "mantle cell" lymphoma) +/– polyposis
	5. Follicular centroblastic-centrocytic lymphoma
	6. Plasmacytic lymphoma
T-cell types	
	Peripheral T-cell lymphomas (pleomorphic, small, medium-sized or large, immunoblastic, large cell anaplastic, undefined)
	+/– Enteropathy
	+/– Eosinophilia

3.1.2 KIEL, 17–19 FEBRUARY 1988

A panel composed of members of the ELC (Diebold, Rilke, Wright, Kapançi, the designated secretary Pallesen, and myself) met to prepare the first meeting of the proposed society.

3.1.3 21 MARCH 1988

Kapançi sent a letter to all the members of the ELC and enclosed a copy of the constitution that had been reviewed by a lawyer. The most important issue was the name. The lawyer thought that the term "Association" should be used instead of "Society" on legal grounds. Kapançi sent the final document to Rilke, Wright, Diebold, and myself to be signed. Kapançi also signed it because he was a resident of Geneva, which was the place where the Association was officially founded.

3.2 GENEVA, 11–15 APRIL 1988

The **first meeting** of the **European Association for Haematopatholgy (EAHP)** was organized by KAPANÇI with the aid of an outside organization (Symporg A.G.). The programme was prepared by an "interim EAHP committee" formed by the ELC. The number of registered participants totalled 246. They came from 20 European countries: France (33), West Germany (33), Italy (31), Switzerland (20), United Kingdom (19), Belgium (16), Denmark (14), Spain (14), Austria (10), The Netherlands (8), Sweden (7), Yugoslavia (6), Norway (4), Poland (4), Portugal (4), Hungary (3), Turkey (3), Finland (1), Monaco (1), and Czechoslovakia (1). There were also participants from the USA (5), Israel (5), Canada (2), Hong Kong (1) and China (1). The latter was YAN QUING-HAN from Beijing, who presented us with a drawing of the Chinese symbol for the current year (a dragon) as a sign of luck.

In my introductory remarks as proposed president I gave a short history of the EAHP. The Association was formed in several phases. The first step was the founding of the ELC in 1974, which started with eight members from various European countries. The ELC met regularly to discuss the development and further refinement of the Kiel classification of NHL. In 1982 the ELSG was founded to offer and promote training in the diagnosis of NHL according to the Kiel classification. The Study Group had organized four workshops for about 100 participants from almost all European countries. At the most recent workshop two guests had been invited from the USA (HARRIS and BANKS). The workshops were to continue under the responsibility of the EAHP.

There were four parts to the programme of the meeting:

1. **Tutorial** for trainees in haematopathology. This offering was overbooked. Slide sets were distributed to a total of 120 participants. The chairman was WRIGHT. The topics of the tutorial were: reactive and inflammatory conditions of the lymphoreticular system (F. LEE), Hodgkin's disease and related conditions (WRIGHT), B-cell NHL (I. LAUDER), T-cell NHL (STANSFELD), and extranodal lymphomas (K. MCLENNAN).
2. **Scientific sessions with symposia**. There were 28 invited speakers. A keynote lecture was given by MAK (of Toronto) entitled "The Immunoglobulin Gene Superfamily". There were 16 proffered papers. A **round table conference** on B-cell lymphomas of the digestive tract was moderated by MÜLLER-HERMELINK. The participants (ISAACSON, SCHMID, RADASZKIEWICZ, P.M. KLUIN, P. MOUBAYED, and myself) came to conclusion that MALT lymphomas of the gastrointestinal tract represent a new entity. The American participants were surprised that the members of the ELC (including myself) stood solidly behind ISAACSON.

This was probably the most important message of the first meeting of the EAHP.

The topics of the **symposia** were: "New Approaches to the Study of Lymphomas" (chairpersons: HARRIS and MASON), "Hodgkin's Lymphomas and the Borderline to Non-Hodgkin's Lymphomas" (chairpersons: MIODUSZEWSKA and BANKS), and "Malignant Lymphomas of the Mucosa-Associated Lymphatic Tissue (MALT)" (chairmen: HEIMANN and WIDGREN).

The **proffered papers** were presented in two sessions entitled "News about NHL and Related Topics" (chairmen: C.D. BARONI and DIEBOLD) and "Histopathology of Bone Marrow and Spleen" (chairmen: GEORGII and NÉZELOF).

3. **Workshop** on "Extranodal Lymphomas". 78 cases were presented and then discussed after slides had been examined under the microscope. The chairman was SCHWARZE and the panelists were DIEBOLD, FELLER, ISAACSON, STANSFELD, and myself.
4. **Poster Session**. The reviewers were BÜRKI and VAN UNNIK.

None of the presentations were published in detail. LAUDER and WRIGHT, however, gave a report on the meeting in »Haematological Oncology« [98]. The secretary of the EAHP, PALLESEN (Fig. 20), wrote in his report in November 1988: "There was a feeling that the general level of this first meeting was high. Probably, the program was slightly overloaded leaving very short time for other useful activities (private meetings etc.)."

The first **business meeting** of the EAHP was held on 13 April. The chairman was WRIGHT. At this meeting the Constitution worked out by the "interim committee" was officially confirmed. The aims of the EAHP were stated in the Constitution as follows:

"Article 2: Aims

The purpose of this Association shall be to further the study of diseases of the haematopoietic and lymphoreticular systems and to promote the exchange and dissemination of knowledge concerning the diagnosis and treatment of diseases through:

1. The stimulation of interest, investigation, exchange and dissemination of knowledge concerning haematopathology.
2. Coordination and integration of the morphological aspect of haematopathology with other allied aspects.
3. Promotion of research on haematopathology.
4. Organisation of meetings, workshops and tutorials."

The following officers were elected at the meeting. The executive committee was made up of three officers (president: myself; president-elect: WRIGHT;

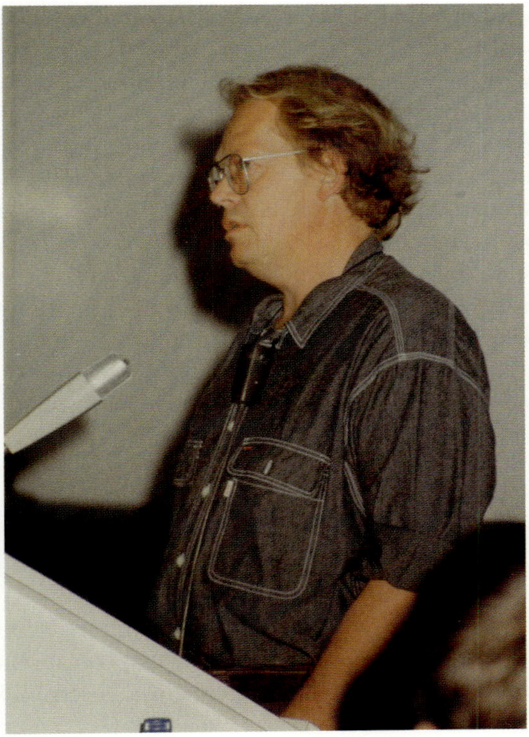

Fig. 20 G. PALLESEN, first secretary of the European Association for Haematopathology

secretary-treasurer: PALLESEN) and six councillors (F. DELACRETAZ, DIEBOLD, KELÉNYI, MASON, MORAGAS, and RILKE). ROBB-SMITH was elected as an honorary member. WRIGHT proposed that I be appointed as "honorary president for life" and this was accepted.

Plans for the next two meetings of the EAHP were also discussed. It was decided that the next meeting would be held in conjunction with the European Society of Pathology in Porto, Portugal, 2–9 September 1989. Negotiations were started with the president of the European Society of Pathology, LLOMBART-BOSCH, who was also a member of the EAHP and was in attendance at the meeting in Geneva. Further meetings were held in 1988 to prepare the final programme. Besides the presidents of the involved societies (LLOMBART-BOSCH, D. SERRAO, and M. SOBRIÑHO-SIMOES) MARIA CLARA SAMBADE would be of great help in organizing the meeting in Porto. She was well trained in lymphoma pathology and took great interest in the Association.

The third meeting would be held in Würzburg in 1990 and was to be organized by MÜLLER-HERMELINK.

YAN brought a greeting to all members of the EAHP from Chinese pathologists. He reported briefly on the "Chinese Lymphoma Research and Cooperation Association" that had held its first meeting in 1977. He also addressed an open invitation to the members of the EAHP to their next meeting in the autumn of 1989 in Fu-Chou on the southeast coast of China.

ROBB-SMITH had sent a telegram from the UK that, unfortunately, was not read aloud. The telegram was addressed to me and the Association and said: "Congratulations inaugural meeting. Regret absence. You are lighting flambeau d'Hematologie. Gesundheit. R.-S."

3.3 PORTO, PORTUGAL, 6–7 SEPTEMBER 1989

At the **second meeting of the EAHP** there were three symposia on 6 September: "Myelodysplastic Syndrome (Preleukemia)" organized by GEORGII, "New Approaches in the Study of Lymphomas" organized by MASON, "Hodgkin's Disease" organized by STEIN, and "T-Cell Lymphomas" organized by myself.

On 7 September there was a slide seminar on "Histopathology of the Spleen" organized by DIEBOLD, H. J. STUTTE, and J. VAN KRIEKEN. At a joint meeting with the European Society of Pathology ISAACSON gave a lecture on "Malignant Lymphomas of the Mucosa Associated Lymphatic Tissue (MALT Lymphomas)".

4 EPILOGUE, 1989–2004

The EAHP has had 11 meetings since the first one in Geneva (see p. 119). The most recent one was held in Thessaloniki, Greece. It was organized by PAPADIMITRIOU. The number of participants had risen to 509, which was more than double the number (246) attending the first meeting in Geneva. They came from all continents. The pathology of the bone marrow was more at the focus of attention, whereas lymphomas had been in the foreground at the first meeting.

At first the Kiel classification was used by all members of the EAHP. This changed at the seventh meeting in Toledo, Spain, in 1994, which took place shortly after the so-called REAL classification ("revised European-American lymphoma classification") had been suggested by an international group at the proposal of ISAACSON and STEIN [99]. In this classification the updated Kiel classification was revised in a few places and the previously excluded extranodal lymphomas were added. Hodgkin's lymphomas were also included. At the request of the Editor of »Histopathology« I wrote a comment on the classification [100] in which I emphasized how important the initiative of ISAACSON and STEIN on the European side and of HARRIS and JAFFE on the American side was for improving the ever so crucial transatlantic communication.

At the meeting in Toledo, after much discussion, it was decided that a generally acceptable and binding classification should be developed on the basis of the REAL classification. Members of both the Society for Hematopathology and the EAHP should get together and come to an agreement which would be published as a "Blue Book" by the WHO.

At the initiative of J. O. ARMITAGE, however, the clinical value of the Working Formulation in comparison with the Kiel classification and the REAL classification would be investigated beforehand. An international panel of experienced haematopathologists did a study at several institutions in various countries. The results were first presented just orally by ROSENBERG at a meeting in Omaha, NE, USA on 11 September 1997. His presentation was very fair. He reported that the Working Formulation, in which he had invested so much time and energy, was clearly inferior in clinical value to both the Kiel and the REAL classifications. The latter were of equal value and clinically useful. The results were also discussed at a meeting at Airlie House in November 1997 [101]. At that meeting the members of a "clinical advisory committee" came to a unanimous agreement that a "Blue Book" should be published by the WHO. After further protracted discussions, what became known as the WHO classification (II) was finally published in 2001 [102] in the new series organized by the UICC in Lyon under the direction of P. Kleihues.

The publication of the new WHO classification eased the tension. It was not received with enthusiasm by all clinicians, however, as is the fate of many new classifications. The WHO classification is now undergoing scrutiny. Inevitably though, another new classification based on new criteria or new methods will be introduced in a few years. As Rappaport so rightly cited the old Viennese words of wisdom: Everything is just a transition!

REFERENCES

1 Maximow AA (1927) Blut und blutbildende Organe. In: Stöhr P, von Möllendorff W (eds) Handbuch der mikroskopischen Anatomie des Menschen, vol 1, part 1. Springer, Berlin, pp 232–583

2 Naegeli O (1931) Blutkrankheiten und Blutdiagnostik. 5th edn. Springer, Berlin

3 Block MH (1976) Text-atlas of hematology. Lea & Fiebiger, Philadelphia

4 Wienbeck J (1942) Die menschliche Leukämie und die leukämoiden Veränderungen. Fischer, Jena

5 Lennert K (1942) Zur Praxis der pathologisch-anatomischen Knochenmarksuntersuchung. Frankf Z Pathol 63:267–299

6 Lennert K, Feller AC (1992) Histopathology of non-Hodgkin's lymphomas (based on the updated Kiel classification). 2nd edn. Springer, New York Berlin Heidelberg, p 264

7 Hui PK, Feller AC, Lennert K (1988) High-grade non-Hodgkin's lymphoma of B-cell type. I. Histopathology. Histopathology 12:127–143

8 Dorfman RF (1994) Hematopathology: a crescendo of scholar activity. Maude Abbott Lecture. Modern Pathology 7:226–241

9 Wintrobe MM (1985) Hematology, the blossoming of a science. A story of inspiration and effort. Lea & Fiebiger, Philadelphia

10 Rappaport H (1966) Tumors of the hematopoietic system. Atlas of tumor pathology, sect 3, fasc 8. Armed Forces Institute of Pathology, Washington DC

11 Lukes RJ, Collins RD (1992) Tumors of the hematopoietic system. Atlas of tumor pathology, second series, fasc 28. Armed Forces Institute of Pathology, Washington DC

12 Robb-Smith AHT (1947) The lymph node biopsy. In: Dyke SC (ed) Recent advances in clinical pathology. J & A Churchill, London, pp 350–370

13 Symmers WStC (1978) The lymphoreticular system. In: Symmers WStC (ed) Systemic pathology, 2nd edn, vol 2. Churchill Livingstone, Edinburgh London New York, pp 504–891

14 The Japan Society of the RES, Editorial Office (ed) (1961) The first general meeting in Sendai, June 26, 1961. Proceedings of the Japan Society of the Reticulo-Endothelial System, vol 1

15 Rüttimann A (ed) (1967) Progress in lymphology. Thieme, Stuttgart

16 Lukes RJ (1967) A review of the American concept of malignant lymphoma. The evolution of a modern classification. In: Rüttimann A (ed) Progress in lymphology. Thieme, Stuttgart, pp 109–119

17 Gall EA, Mallory TB (1942) Malignant lymphoma. A clinico-pathologic survey of 618 cases. Am J Pathol 18:381–429

18 Rappaport H (1964) The histologic aspects of malignant lymphoreticular neoplasms. In: Roulet FC (ed) Symposium on lymphoreticular tumours in Africa, Paris, 1963. Karger, Basel New York, pp 174–210

19 Lennert K (1967) Classification of malignant lymphomas (European concept). In: Rüttimann A (ed) Progress in lymphology. Thieme, Stuttgart, pp 103–109

20 Robb-Smith AHT (1964) Introduction: The classification and natural history of the lymphadenopathies. In: Pack GT, Ariel IM (eds) Lymphomas and related diseases. Treatment of cancer and allied diseases, vol 9. Hoeber Medical Divistion, Harper & Row, New York, pp 1–27

21 Mathé G, Rappaport H, O'Conor GT, Torloni H (1976) Histological and cytological typing of neoplastic diseases of haematopoietic and lymphoid tissues. International histological classification of tumors, no 14. World Health Organization, Geneva

22 Lennert K (1971) Follicular lymphoma: a special entity of malignant lymphomas. In: Plenary session papers. 1. Meeting of the European Division of the International Society of Haematology, Milano, 1971. Arti Grafiche Fratelli Ferrari, Milano, pp 109–122

23 Lennert K (1973) Follicular lymphoma. A tumor of the germinal centers. In: Akazaki K, Rappaport H, Berard CW, Bennett JM, Ishikawa E (eds) Malignant diseases of the hematopoietic system. GANN monograph on cancer research, vol 15. University of Tokyo Press, Tokyo, pp 217–231

24 Lennert K, Niedorf HR (1969) Nachweis von desmosomal verknüpften Reticulumzellen im follikulären Lymphom (Brill-Symmers). Virchows Arch [B] 4:148–150

25 Liao KT, Rosai J, Daneshbod K (1972) Malignant histiocytosis with cutaneous involvement and eosinophilia. Am J Clin Pathol 57:438–448

26 Knecht H, Lennert K (1981) Vorgeschichte und klinisches Bild der lymphogranulomatosis X (einschließlich [angio]immunoblastischer Lymphadenopathie). Schweiz Med Wochenschr 111:1108–1121

27 Knecht H, Lennert K (1981) Verlauf, Therapie und maligne Transformation der Lymphogranulomatosis X (einschließlich [angio]immunoblastischer Lymphadenopathie). Schweiz Med Wochenschr 111:1122–1130

28 Frizzera G, Moran EM, Rappaport H (1974) Angio-immunoblastic lymphadenopathy with dysproteinemа. Lancet i:1070–1073

29 Shimoyama MK, Tobinai K, Minato K, Watanabe S (1982) Immunoblastic lymphadenopathy (IBL)-like T-cell lymphoma. GANN monograph on cancer research, vol 28. University of Tokyo Press, Tokyo, pp 121–134

30 Nowell PC (1960) Phytohemagglutinin: an initiator of mitosis in cultures of normal human leukocytes. Cancer Res 20:462–466

31 Stein H, Lennert K, Parwaresch MR (1972) Malignant lymphomas of B-cell type. Lancet ii: 855–857

32 Stein H, Kaiserling E, Lennert K (1973) Neue Gesichtspunkte zur Systematik maligner Lymphome auf dem Boden immunchemischer Analysen. In: Stacher A (ed) Leukämien und maligne Lymphome. Urban & Schwarzenberg, München Berlin Wien, pp 195–201

33 Diebold J, Zittoun R, Fine JM, Tricot G, Camilleri JP, Simon F, Alcalay M, Bousser J (1971) Syndrome lymphoprolifératif avec production de macroglobuline IgM purement intracellulaire. Nouv Rev franc Hémat 11:429–433

34 Kaiserling E, Stein H, Lennert K (1973) IgM-producing malignant lymphomas without macroglobulinemia. Morphological and immunochemical findings. Virchows Arch [B] 14:1–18

35 Good RA (1965) Personal communication

36 Brittinger G, Bartels H, Bremer K, Burger A, Dühmke E, Gunzer U, König E, Stacher A, Stein H, Theml H, Waldner R (Kieler Lymphomgruppe) (1977) Retrospektive Untersuchungen zur klinischen Bedeutung der Kiel-Klassifikation der malignen Non-Hodgkin-Lymphome. Strahlentherapie 153:222–228

37 Bremer K (1981) Kiel classification of non-Hodgkin's lymphomas: data of a retrospective analysis and preliminary results of a prospective multicenter trial. In: Progress in lymphology. Proceedings of the 7th International Congress of Lymphology, Florence, 1979. Avicenum Czechoslovak Medical Press, Prague, pp 303–306

38 Brittinger G, Bartels H, Common H, Dühmke E, Fülle HH, Gunzer U, Gyenes T, Heinz R, König E, Meusers P, Paukstat M, Pralle H, Theml H, Köpcke W, Thieme C, Zwingers T, Musshoff K, Stacher A, Brücher H, Herrmann F, Ludwig WD, Pribilla W, Burger-Schüler A, Löhr GW, Gremmel H, Oertel J, Gerhartz H, Koeppen K-M, Boll I, Huhn D, Binder T, Schoengen A, Nowicki L, Pees HW, Scheurlen PG, Leopold H, Wannenmacher M, Schmidt M, Löffler H, Michlmayr G, Thiel E, Zettel R, Rühl U, Wilke HJ, Schwarze E-W, Stein H, Feller AC, Lennert K (Kiel Lymphoma Study Group) (1984) Clinical and prognostic relevance of the Kiel classification of non-Hodgkin lymphomas: results of a prospective multicenter study by the Kiel Lymphoma Study Group. Hematol Oncol 2:269–306

39 Stein H, Lennert K, Parwaresch MR (1972) Malignant lymphomas of B-cell type. Lancet ii:855–857

40 Lennert K, Stein H, Kaiserling E (1975) Cytological and functional criteria for the classification of malignant lymphomata. Br J Cancer 31 [Suppl ii]:29–43

41 Lennert K, Stein H, Kaiserling E (1974) New criteria for the classification of malignant lymphomas. In: Líbanský J, Donner L (eds) Present problems in haematology. Excerpta Medica, Amsterdam, pp 113–119

42 Peckham MJ (ed) (1975) Non-Hodgkin's lymphomata. Br J Cancer 31 [Suppl ii]

43 Lukes RJ, Collins RD (1975) New approaches to the classification of the lymphomata. Br J Cancer 31 [Suppl ii]:1–28

44 Lennert K (1961) Lymphknoten. Diagnostik in Schnitt und Ausstrich. Cytologie und Lymphadenitis. In: Lubarsch O, Henke F, Rössle R, Uehlinger E (eds) Handbuch der speziellen pathologischen Anatomie und Histologie, vol 1, part 3A. Springer, Berlin Göttingen Heidelberg

45 Gérard-Marchant R, Hamlin I, Lennert K, Rilke F, Stansfeld AG, van Unnik JAM (1974) Classification of non-Hodgkin's lymphomas. [Letter to the Editor] Lancet ii:406–408

46 Bennett MH, Farrer-Brown G, Henry K, Jelliffe AM (1974) Classification of non-Hodgkin's lymphomas. [Letter to the Editor] Lancet ii:405–406

47 Dorfman RF (1974) Classification of non-Hodgkin's lymphomas. [Letter to the Editor] Lancet i:1295–1296
48 Kay HEM (1974) Classification of non-Hodgkin's lymphomas. [Letter to the Editor] Lancet ii:586
49 Lennert K (1975) Morphology and classification of malignant lymphomas and so-called reticuloses. In: Jellinger K, Seitelberger F (eds) Malignant lymphomas of the nervous system. Acta neuropath (Berlin) 6 [Suppl]:1–16
50 Jellinger K, Radaszkiewicz T (1976) Involvement of the central nervous system in malignant lymphoma. Virchows Arch [A] 370:345–362
51 Lennert K, Mohri N, Stein H, Kaiserling E (1975) The histopathology of malignant lymphoma. Br J Haematol 31 [Suppl]:193–203
52 Lennert K (1976) Klassifikation und Morphologie der Non-Hodgkin-Lymphome. In: Löffler H (ed) Maligne Lymphome und monoklonale Gammopathien. Hämatologie und Bluttransfusion, vol 18. Lehmanns, München, pp 145–166
53 Stein H (1976) Immunchemische und immunzytochemische Befunde bei Non-Hodgkin-Lymphomen. In: Löffler H (ed) Maligne Lymphome und monoklonale Gammopathien. Hämatologie und Bluttransfusion, vol 18. Lehmanns, München, pp 167–183
54 Kaiserling E (1976) Elektronenmikroskopische Befunde bei Non-Hodgkin-Lymphomen. In: Löffler H (ed) Maligne Lymphome und monoklonale Gammopathien. Hämatologie und Bluttransfusion, vol 18. Lehmanns, München, pp 185–198
55 Mandard AM, Tanguy A, Vernhes JC, Abbatucci JS, Mandard JC (1977) Lymphomes malins non hodgkiniens. Étude rétrospective de 64 cas classés selon les nomenclatures de Kiel et Rappaport. Bull Cancer (Paris) 64:347–364
56 Meugé-Moraw C, Hoerni B, de Mascarel A, Durand M, Richaud P, Hoerni-Simon G, Chauvergne J, Lagarde C (1978) Non-Hodgkin malignant lymphomas. Clinicopathologic correlations with the Kiel classification. Retrospective analysis of a series of 274 cases. Eur J Cancer 14:587–592
57 Lennert K, Kaiserling E, Müller-Hermelink HK (1978) Malignant lymphomas: models of differentiation and cooperation of lymphoreticular cells. In: Clarkson B, Marks PA, Till JE (eds) Differentiation of normal and neoplastic hematopoietic cells, book B. Cold Spring Harbor conferences on cell proliferation, vol 5. Cold Spring Harbor Laboratory, Cold Spring Harbor, pp 897–913
58 Lennert K in collaboration with Mohri N, Stein H, Kaiserling E, Müller-Hermelink (1978) Malignant lymphomas other than Hodgkin's disease. Handbuch der speziellen pathologischen Anatomie und Histologie, vol 1, part 3B. Springer, Berlin Heidelberg New York
59 Lukes RJ, Parker JW, Taylor CR, Tindle BH, Cramer AD, Lincoln TL (1978) Immunologic approach to non-Hodgkin lymphomas and related leukemias. Analysis of the results of multiparameter studies of 425 cases. Semin Hematol 15:322–351
60 Lennert K in collaboration with Stein H (1981) Histopathology of non-Hodgkin's lymphomas (based on the Kiel classification). Springer, Berlin Heidelberg New York

61 Stansfeld AG (1985) Lymphomas. In: Stansfeld AG (ed) Lymph node biopsy interpretation. Churchill Livingstone, Edinburgh London New York, pp 228–329

62 Nathwani BN (1979) A critical analysis of the classifications of non-Hodgkin's lymphomas. Cancer 44:347–384

63 Banks PM, Chan J, Cleary ML, Delsol G, De Wolf-Peeters C, Gatter K, Grogan TM, Harris NL, Isaacson PG, Jaffe ES, Mason DY, Pileri S, Ralfkiaer E, Stein H, Warnke RA (1992) Mantle cell lymphoma: a proposal for unification of morphologic, immunologic and molecular data. Am J Surg Pathol 16:637–640

64 Swerdlow SH, Williams ME (2002) From centrocytic to mantle cell lymphoma: a clinicopathologic and molecular review of 3 decades. Hum Pathol 33:7–20

65 Gödde-Salz E, Schwarze E-W, Stein H, Lennert K, Grote W (1981) Cytogenetic findings in T-zone lymphoma. J Cancer Res Clin Oncol 101:81–89

66 Gahrton G, Juliusson G, Robert KH, Friberg K, Zech L (1985) Chromosomal aberrations in leukemic low-grade malignant B-cell lymphoproliferative neoplasias. In: Proceedings of the second international conference on malignant lymphomas, Lugano, 1985. Martinus Nijhoff, Boston, pp 81–87

67 Fifth International Workshop on Chromosomes in Leukemia-Lymphoma (1987) Correlation of chromosome abnormalities with histologic and immunologic characteristics in non-Hodgkin's lymphoma and adult T cell leukemia-lymphoma. Blood 70:1554–1564

68 O'Connor NTJ, Wainscoat JS, Weatherall DJ, Gatter KC, Feller AC, Isaacson P, Jones D, Lennert K, Pallesen G, Ramsey A, Stein H, Wright DH, Mason DY (1985) Rearrangement of the T-cell receptor β-chain gene in the diagnosis of lymphoproliferative disorders. Lancet i:1295–1297

69 Griesser H, Feller A, Lennert K, Minden M, Mak TW (1986) Rearrangement of the β chain of the T cell antigen receptor and immunoglobulin genes in lymphoproliferative disorders. J Clin Invest 78:1179–1184

70 Chadli A, Lennert K (1979) Les lymphomas malins non-hodgkiniens du tube digestif. Ann Anat Pathol 24:231–250

71 Delarue J (1963) Louis Fruhling. Ann d'Anat Pathol 8:7–14

72 Musshoff K, Schmidt-Vollmer H, Lennert K, Sandritter W (1976) Preliminary clinical findings on the Kiel classificaiton of malignant lymphomas. Z Krebsforsch 87:229–238

73 Mathé G, Seligmann M, Tubiana M (eds) (1978) Lymphoid neoplasias I. Recent results in cancer research, vol 64. Springer, Berlin Heidelberg New York

74 Lennert K, Stein H (1978) Personal points of view on the Kiel classification. In: Mathé G, Seligmann M, Tubiana M (eds) Lymphoid neoplasias I. Recent results in cancer research, vol 64. Springer, Berlin Heidelberg New York, pp 31–37

75 Levy R, Kaplan HS (eds) (1978) Malignant lymphoma. UICC technical report series, vol 37. UICC, Geneva

76 The Non-Hodgkin's Lymphoma Pathologic Classification Project (1982) National Cancer Institute sponsored study of classifications of non-Hodgkin's lymphomas. Summary and description of a Working Formulation for clinical usage. Cancer 49:2112–2135

77 Nathwani BN, Metter GE, Gams RA, Bartolucci AA, Hartsock RJ, Neiman RS, Byrne GE, Barcos M, Kim H, Rappaport H (1983) Malignant lymphoma, mixed cell type, diffuse. Blood 62:200–208

78 Lennert K, Collins RD, Lukes RJ (1983) Concordance of the Kiel and Lukes-Collins classifications of non-Hodgkin's lymphomas. Histopathology 7:549–559

79 Knapp W (ed) (1981) Leukemia markers. Academic, London

80 Cabanne F, Bonenfant JL (eds) (1980) Anatomie pathologique: principes de pathologie générale et spéciale. Les Presses de l'Université Laval, Québec, and Maloine, Paris

81 Vitetta ES (ed) (1982) B and T cell tumors. UCLA symposia on molecular and cellular biology, vol 24. Academic, New York London

82 Lennert K, Stein H, Feller AC, Gerdes J (1982) Morphology, cytochemistry, and immunohistology of T-cell lymphomas. In: Vitetta ES (ed) B and T cell tumors. UCLA symposia on molecular and cellular biology, vol 24. Academic, New York London, pp 9–28

83 Gajl-Peczalska KJ, Bloomfield CD, Frizzera G, Kersey JH, Lebien TW (1982) Diversity of phenotypes of non-Hodgkin's malignant lymphoma. In: Vitetta ES (ed) B and T cell tumors. UCLA symposia on molecular and cellular biology, vol 24. Academic, New York London, pp 63–68

84 Hanaoka M, Shirakawa S, Yodoi J, Uchiyama T, Takatsuki K (1979) Adult T cell leukemia. Histological features of the lymphoid tissues. In: Müller-Ruchholtz W, Müller-Hermelink HK (eds) Function and structure of the immune system. Advances in experimental medicine and biology, vol 144. Plenum, New York, pp 613–621

85 Lennert K, Schwarze E-W (1983) Malignant lymphomas of the head and neck. In: Rhys Evans PH, Robin PE, Fielding JWL (eds) Head and neck cancer. Castle House Publications, Tunbridge Wells, pp 81–88

86 Lennert K, Hübner K (ed) (1983) Hämatopathologie. Verhandlungen der Deutschen Gesellschaft für Pathologie, vol 67. Fischer, Jena

87 Lennert K, Kikuchi M, Sato E, Suchi T, Stansfeld AG, Feller AC, Hansmann M-L, Müller-Hermelink HK, Gödde-Salz E (1985) HTLV-positive and -negative T-cell lymphomas. Morphological and immunohistochemical differences between European and HTLV-positive Japanese T-cell lymphomas. Int J Cancer 35:65–72

88 Takatsuki K, Uchiyama T, Sagawa K, Yodoi J (1976) Adult T cell leukemia in Japan. Excerpta Medica Int Congr Ser 415:73–77

89 Bardwick PA, Zvaifler NJ, Gill GN, Newman D, Greenway GD, Resnick DL (1980) Plasma cell dyscrasia with polyneuropathy, organomegaly, endocrinopathy, M-protein, and skin changes: the POEMS syndrome. Medicine 59:311–322

90 Griesser H, Feller AC, Mak TW, Lennert K (1987) Clonal rearrangements of T-cell receptor and immunoglobulin genes and immunophenotypic antigen expression in different subclasses of Hodgkin's disease. Int J Cancer 40:157–160

91 Suchi T, Lennert K, Tu LY, Kikuchi M, Sato E, Stansfeld AG, Feller AC (1987) Histopathology and immunohistochemistry of peripheral T cell lymphomas: a proposal for their classification. J Clin Pathol 40:995–1015

92 Berard CW, Dorfman RF, Kaufman N (eds) (1987) Malignant lymphoma. IAP monographs in pathology, no 29. Williams and Wilkins, Baltimore

93 Dorfman RF (1987) Introduction. In: Berard CW, Dorfman RF, Kaufman N (eds) Malignant lymphoma. IAP monographs in pathology, no 29. Williams and Wilkins, Baltimore, pp 1–7
94 Nathwani BN (1987) Classifying non-Hodgkin's lymphomas. In: Berard CW, Dorfman RF, Kaufman N (eds) Malignant lymphoma. Monographs in pathology, no 29. Williams and Wilkins, Baltimore, pp 18–80
95 Lennert K (spec ed) (1981) Symposium on recent data from the characterization of malignant lymphoma. J Cancer Res 101:1
96 The Nationwide Lymphoma Pathology Cooperative Group (NLPCG) (1985) A retrospective histological study of malignant lymphoma in China using the NLPCG classification. Jpn J Clin Oncol 15:645–651
97 Isaacson PG, Norton AJ (1994) Extranodal lymphomas. Churchill Livingstone, Edinburgh London New York
98 Lauder I, Wright D (1989) Foundation meeting of the European Association for Haematopathology. Haematol Oncol 7:319–323
99 Harris NL, Jaffe ES, Stein H, Banks PM, Chan JKC, Cleary ML, Delsol G, De Wolf-Peeters C, Falini B, Gatter KC, Grogan TM, Isaacson PG, Knowles DM, Mason DY, Müller-Hermelink H-K, Pileri SA, Piris MA, Ralfkiaer E, Warnke RA (1994) A revised European-American classification of lymphoid neoplasms: a proposal from the International Lymphoma Study Group. Blood 84:1361–1392
100 Lennert K (1995) The proposal of a revised European-American lymphoma classification – a new start of a transatlantic discussion. Histopathology 26:481–483
101 Harris NL, Jaffe ES, Diebold J, Flandrin G, Müller-Hermelink HK, Vardiman J, Lister TA, Bloomfield CD (1999) World Health Organization classification of neoplastic diseases of the hematopoietic and lymphoid tissues: report of the Clinical Advisory Committee meeting – Airlie House, Virginia, November 1997. J Clin Oncol 17:3835–3849
102 Jaffe ES, Harris NL, Stein H, Vardiman JW (eds) (2001) Pathology and genetics of tumours of haematopoietic and lymphoid tissue. World Health Organization classification of tumours. IARC Press, Lyon

Printing: Krips bv, Meppel
Binding: Stürtz, Würzburg